MOBILITIES AND HE

Geographies of Health

Series Editors
Allison Williams, Associate Professor, School of Geography and Earth
Sciences, McMaster University, Canada
Susan Elliott, Dean of the Faculty of Social Sciences,
McMaster University, Canada

There is growing interest in the geographies of health and a continued interest in what has more traditionally been labeled medical geography. The traditional focus of 'medical geography' on areas such as disease ecology, health service provision and disease mapping (all of which continue to reflect a mainly quantitative approach to inquiry) has evolved to a focus on a broader, theoretically informed epistemology of health geographies in an expanded international reach. As a result, we now find this subdiscipline characterized by a strongly theoretically-informed research agenda, embracing a range of methods (quantitative; qualitative and the integration of the two) of inquiry concerned with questions of: risk; representation and meaning; inequality and power; culture and difference, among others. Health mapping and modeling has simultaneously been strengthened by the technical advances made in multilevel modeling, advanced spatial analytic methods and GIS, while further engaging in questions related to health inequalities, population health and environmental degradation.

This series publishes superior quality research monographs and edited collections representing contemporary applications in the field; this encompasses original research as well as advances in methods, techniques and theories. The *Geographies of Health* series will capture the interest of a broad body of scholars, within the social sciences, the health sciences and beyond.

Also in the series

Space, Place and Mental Health
Sarah Curtis
ISBN 978 0 7546 7331 6

Healing Waters
Therapeutic Landscapes in Historic and Contemporary Ireland
Ronan Foley
ISBN 978 0 7546 7652 2

Towards Enabling Geographies:
'Disabled' Bodies and Minds in Society and Space
Edited by Vera Chouinard, Edward Hall, and Robert Wilton
ISBN 978 0 7546 7561 7

Mobilities and Health

ANTHONY C. GATRELL
Lancaster University, UK

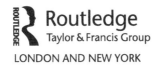

Routledge
Taylor & Francis Group

LONDON AND NEW YORK

First published 2011 by Ashgate Publishing

Published 2016 by Routledge
2 Park Square, Milton Park, Abingdon, Oxfordshire OX14 4RN
711 Third Avenue, New York, NY 10017, USA

First issued in paperback 2016

Routledge is an imprint of the Taylor & Francis Group, an informa business

British Library Cataloguing in Publication Data
Gatrell, Anthony C.
  Mobilities and health. -- (Ashgate's geographies of health
  series)
  1. Medical geography. 2. Epidemiology.
  I. Title II. Series III. Gatrell, Tony.
  614.4'2-dc22

Library of Congress Cataloging-in-Publication Data
Gatrell, Anthony C.
  Mobilities and health / by Anthony C. Gatrell.
    p. cm. -- (Ashgate's geographies of health series)
  Includes bibliographical references and index.
  ISBN 978-1-4094-1992-1 (hardback)
1. Medical geography. 2. Environmental health. 3. Social medicine. I. Title. II. Series:
Ashgate's geographies of health series.
  [DNLM: 1. Travel. 2. Epidemiology. 3. Geography. 4. Residence Characteristics. 5.
Sociology, Medical. WA 108]

  RA792.G384 2011
  614.4'2--dc23

                                                                        2011017634

  ISBN 13: 978-1-138-26923-1 (pbk)
  ISBN 13: 978-1-4094-1992-1 (hbk)

Contents

For Caroline, Anna, and Emma

List of Figures

List of Tables

Preface

When we think about our health and well-being, or about our consumption of health services and medical care, we often reflect on how these are shaped by the places or areas we live in, or have lived in. Both academic studies and the popular press stress that our health, our exposure to disease risk factors, our life expectancy, and so on, are shaped by 'place'. When we think about our well-being, we call to mind those places – some perhaps exotic, others quite ordinary – that have added to our sense of well-ness. Equally, when we consume health care we invariably do so by visiting a health centre or hospital that is physically located some*where*. Whether we are concerned with health outcomes or service locations, we usually have in mind places or areas with *fixed* geographical locations and boundaries.

Against this notion of 'fixity' we can set a growing contemporary concern with things that are mobile and fluid. It is the connections between movement, or mobility, and health that I want to excavate and illustrate in this book. Studying relationships between population movement (usually focusing on migration) and human health, and our understanding of the geographic spread of disease, have long been the concerns of epidemiologists and geographers. Here, I want to expand the range of study to include a much wider set of issues that are relevant to public health, while not neglecting those important topics. But I do not focus solely on health risk due to mobility, since movements can have positive consequences, including those that derive both from the travel experience itself and at the journey's end.

I structure this overview of mobility and health with reference to four mobility domains: travel; migration; diffusion; and communication and care. Each of these four parts is introduced in turn. But I begin by considering a set of concepts and ideas that help to shape our understanding of mobility and health. These are drawn, broadly speaking, from three primary disciplines – geography; sociology; and epidemiology.

My aim is not to compile an exhaustive compendium of literature relating to movement and health. Thus there are topics and issues that I might have covered, but have not. For example, all sport involves bodily movement of some sort or another, but I do not consider the huge topic of relationships between sport and health (or sports injuries, for that matter). I do not attempt an exploration of mobilities at the scale of the individual body. The movement of bodily fluids is not something I examine here (for a discussion of some of these see Longhurst 2001). Nor do I consider other things that move or flow and impact on health. So I do not examine the risks from mobile cigarette smoke, or mobile hazardous waste, or the global transfer of pollutants, drugs or arms. Since these are all important mobilities in relation to health I cannot claim to be comprehensive here.

In preparing this book I have profited both from reading recent monographs and papers drawn from different disciplines. But I have also enjoyed returning to, or discovering, older literatures. There is a temptation to dismiss some of the latter as 'old-fashioned' or theoretically light. I think this is unfortunate. What I have sought to do is to engage with some contemporary theoretical debates but, where appropriate, to draw on some classic studies to inform those debates. I have also relied, where possible, on high-quality empirical work undertaken by more recent researchers, and on 'meta-analyses' of literature, where these already exist. I hope the references indicate where some of my debts lie.

Within the text I make considerable reference to 'networks'. I have long been interested in the networks of relations that bind together academics from different disciplines and from different places. Over a 35 year period I myself have benefited greatly from these rich connections, and I want to thank the key actors in these webs. So, for intellectual sustenance at different periods I thank (in an approximate degree of temporal significance in my career!) the following geographers, social scientists and epidemiologists who have especially enriched me: Peter Haggett, Andy Cliff, Peter Gould, Martyn Senior, Robin Flowerdew, Andrew Lovett, Peter Diggle, Paul Boyle, Simon Kingham, Jan Rigby, Susan Elliott, and John Urry. For other forms of support, especially in the latter stages of my career, I want to thank in particular Paul and Annette Wellings, Nick and Bren Abercrombie, Bob McKinlay, Gavin Brown, Amelia Hunt and, above all, Caroline Gatrell. Caroline's high intellectual standards inspire all those with whom she is networked academically, while her personal warmth and loyalty endears her to all those connected to her socially. Her loving nature is, of course, felt most keenly by her closest family and I thank her, and our children Anna and Emma, for the best connections of all.

Tony Gatrell
Lancaster, March 2011

Chapter 1
Mobilising Concepts

Introducing geographies of health

This book looks at health and health care in a new way. Rather than focus on the health risks and benefits incurred at fixed locations I investigate such risks and benefits as encountered on the move, moves that might be transient or more enduring. I examine too the provision and utilization of health-related information and care, not at sets of discrete locations but instead as they are produced/delivered and consumed/accessed in mobile settings. The objects of study, or units of analysis, are not therefore primarily places or 'nodes'; rather, they are the flows or relationships *between* such nodes.

The book draws primarily, though not exclusively, on the geography of health and the mobilities 'turn' in sociology. I introduce the former briefly here, and in the next section examine what is understood by mobilities.

As an intellectual enterprise, the study of health geographies has taken off during the last 20 years (Gatrell and Elliott 2009, Brown et al. 2010). As with any such enterprise, the approaches are diverse (hence *geographies*) but the common ground is to understand how space and place shape patterns of health and wellbeing, or ill-health and disease, as well as the production and consumption of healthcare. The field has, to an extent, displaced more traditional concerns with mapping and explaining the distribution of disease at different spatial scales, though for many this remains a prime concern given emerging and re-emerging infections across the globe. But a natural science-based *medical geography* has, to a considerable extent, given way to *health geographies* that assert the primacy of the social and cultural. In a way this mirrors developments in geographies of movement, where predominantly positivistic approaches to the field of transport geography have begun to acknowledge the mobilities turn in sociology (Shaw and Hesse 2010).

It would be a gross over-simplification to suggest that traditional approaches to geographies of health were static, mapping the locations of death and disease across sets of fixed geographic units. Mobility and migration have never been neglected. For example, spatial analysis has long been applied to the study of disease spread, or spatial diffusion. Others have acknowledged that, over their life-courses, people move house, perhaps several times, and one cannot simply explain disease distribution according to place of residence at time of diagnosis. Those interested in disease ecology, in which the reciprocal interactions between humans and their environments are paramount (Learmonth 1988, Meade and Emch 2010), have always understood the importance of population movement. Further, health geographers have also long been concerned with issues of accessibility to health care – the ability or otherwise of people to travel to consume health services (Gatrell and Elliott 2009: Chapter 5).

Nonetheless, it remains the case that many contemporary researchers in health geographies adopt a rather static view of the world, either in their analyses of geographic patterns of wellness or illness, or in their analyses of healthcare production or consumption. A particular theme (Gatrell and Elliott 2009: 61-4) has been to separate out the influence of *context* (what places are like) from the influence of *composition* (what kinds of people live in particular places). But a container-like view of spatial context, in which ill-health is mapped within a set of discrete areal units (such as states or counties in the US), is being challenged, either by those who seek to conceptualise space as continuous rather than discrete or those who see it as relational. Among the latter group Cummins and his colleagues (2007) have made the case well, touching on the kinds of subject matter covered in this book. For example, they are critical of the use of straight-line (Euclidean) distance as a measure of spatial separation, and call for more nuanced accounts of health that recognise the influences from a multiplicity of spatial scales (not merely a geographically-defined 'neighbourhood') and that come from people being embedded within a set of networks. They reject what they see as the false dualism of context and composition.

Although some researchers had previously adopted 'post-positivist' approaches in order to describe and interpret (ill-)health in particular settings, it took a seminal paper by Kearns (1993) to encourage a transformation from medical geography to health geography. This has led to a rich literature on the relationships between human health and the experience of place, literature that has drawn on contemporary social and cultural theory and that uses qualitative rather than quantitative methods. As many of the essays in the landmark collection edited by Brown et al. (2010) suggest, it covers perspectives on disabled and marginalised groups, looks at the different ways in which people provide and access care, and puts *place* rather than *space* at the forefront of enquiry. In engaging with people's experiences of place (which might be woodlands, mountain landscapes, care homes, or other health-care settings, for example) research on what are now called 'emotional geographies' (Davidson et al. 2007) complements more traditional research on access to those facilities which may improve health and well-being.

I draw on these and other ideas from the geography of health. But my main aim is to see that this field of enquiry engages with, and draws inspiration from, studies of the mobility of objects and people: studies which, as I suggest in the next section, have been generating considerable interest and excitement among social scientists (including geographers) over the past few years.

Introducing mobilities

At its most simple, mobility involves displacement – movement between locations (Cresswell 2006: 2). Such locations may be places in geographic space, or they may be points a few centimetres apart (such as the movements I make as I type these words at 9.15 pm on Sunday February 14, 2010). Indeed, Cresswell's highly original and important book makes much of the movements involved in dance, and of early attempts to record, photographically, the moving body. Cresswell seeks to understand the *meanings* involved in such movement. Not for him the abstract fact of movement from A to B; rather, the social implications of the movement itself. He makes an interesting analogy between location (an observed point in space) and movement (also observable), and their equivalents (*place* and *mobility*), the latter both imbued with social content, meaning, and power. His interest in mobility as embodied experience (but, as the sub-title of his book suggests, only in the modern Western world) promises to highlight the ways in which it creates, or alternatively affects adversely, health and well-being. However, as with so much of the mobilities turn in contemporary social science the promise of an examination of these relationships remains largely unrealised. The present book seeks to unpick some of these relationships.

Cresswell contrasts, very neatly, two ways of looking at mobility, which he terms (borrowing from the cultural anthropologist Liisa Malkki) a 'sedentarist metaphysics' and a 'nomadic metaphysics' (see also Adey 2010, Chapter 2). In the former view of the world, mobilities – and those who travel – are seen as things to be avoided, or even as threatening or infused with *risk*; for example, the hobo, the tramp, the refugee and asylum seeker are not to be trusted. Movement is dysfunctional. If people do have to move they should do so in a planned, efficient way; but 'the basic assumption is that things (including people) don't move if they can help it' (Cresswell 2006: 29). Even places run the risk of becoming 'placeless' if they become marked with the stamp of uniformity as a result of endless mobility. In a *nomadic metaphysics*, taking its cue from postmodernist views of the world, mobilities are valued and celebrated as expressions of freedom. 'In this new world, a place such as the airport lounge, once seen as a reprehensible site of placelessness, becomes a contemporary symbol of flow, dynamism, and mobility' (Cresswell 2006: 44-5). Such places (or, for some, non-places) become communities of modern nomads. Some of these modern nomads are part of a 'kinetic elite'; a privileged group of international travellers; others are an underclass, servicing the elite while yet others perhaps revel in their freedoms and subversion of state discipline.

Canzler and his colleagues (2008) argue that mobility and the networks associated with it are features of what sociologists call 'second modernity' or a period of 'reflexive modernization'. Clearly, modes of transport such as rail emerged to enable more rapid movement of goods and people during the industrial revolution ('first modernity', sometimes 'simple' modernity, in which travel tended to be uni-modal). Yet we are now in the midst of a period in which we have to cope with the consequences of rapid technological change (Kesselring 2008). Society has to confront itself with new technologies and the risks associated with these. So, for some, a period of second modernity means living in a 'risk society' (Beck 1992), even a 'world risk society' in which risks of disease, climate change, economic crisis and political conflict stretch across the globe and can have rapid consequences. Kesselring (2008: 78) suggests we live in a *mobile* risk society, where the multiplicity and near-universality of networked flow is conjoined with the complexities of modern life. In second modernity, the archetypical social actors are 'the people who circulate close to the top of the global power pyramid, to whom space matters little and distance is not a bother; people at home in many places but in no one place in particular' (Zygmunt Bauman, cited in Kesselring 2008: 78). Further, while first modernity is – in a sense – contained within the nation-state, second modernity is characterised by a world with more porous borders between states. Mobilities, then, characterise second modernity, as does uncertainty, risk and instability.

Canzler and his colleagues (2008: 2-3) argue that there are three components to mobility: first, *movement* (flows and communications); second, *networks* (both the technical infrastructure but also the social frameworks and networks that make movement and interaction possible); and, third, *motility*, the potential for movement the capacity to move, or the intention to move. I am concerned in this book with *movements* of one kind or another among places, whether real or virtual. I limit myself (as in Adey's introductory text) to spatial or geographical mobility – 'spatial displacement – whether material, electronic or potential' (Adey 2010: 13). Social scientists have for many years looked at mobility in social as well as geographic space; that is to say, movement up or down a social hierarchy. This too of course has health consequences: if social position changes to one's advantage one's health is likely to improve, and vice-versa. But I am not primarily concerned with social position here. I concern myself too with *networks*, since one cannot understand disease spread in contemporary society without an understanding of the networks (material and social) that make such spread possible. Since I am primarily concerned with the relations between movement and health, and the accompanying networks, I do not dwell particularly on the human actor's disposition to move (her '*motility*'), though since movement is socially patterned and the networks are unequally distributed socially I shall certainly touch on issues of inequality.

An important theme in mobilities research is the way in which movement is 'hybrid'; that is, it depends upon the interconnections of humans with objects. In a health context examples include the following, all of which are considered later:

- The spread of disease among humans is dependent upon their mode of travel and is speeded up by the growth in air transport and facilitated by airports and the associated infrastructure that are themselves *im*mobile;
- People travel to access healthcare in other countries, but need the means of transport, and the material resources, to do so, as well as medical technologies;
- People can access healthcare online, but only if they have the ICT infrastructure to do so;
- People are exposed to various risks (pollution, accidents) as a result of their using transport technologies or being impacted by others' use.

Thus, in order to understand the connections between health and mobility, we see that while some things move, others do not. Mobility and immobility exist side by side.

Mobility can take place across very different spatial *scales*. It can be very local, as in a trip to the shops or the short journey to work; this kind of mobility has a particular temporal scale too, in that it occurs during the course of day and does not involve any change in residence (save for the worker who lives away from home during the week). It can operate at a national scale, as when people take vacations or short breaks within a country for the purposes of recreation, or when people migrate to another region within the same country. And, of course, mobility can be trans-national; people take vacations abroad or travel overseas on business, or they may move permanently or semi-permanently to settle abroad, either in relation to work or retirement. Knowles (2010: 375) is critical of the mobilities literature for being 'fixated on long-haul journeys and... less interested in restrained geographies of movement around a neighbourhood'.

I consider movements and health at a variety of spatial scales. People can derive health gains from travelling to very local settings – nearby gardens or parks, for example. They can benefit from vacations taken 'at home' (meaning, without going overseas) or they can seek sun, snow and pleasures of different kinds in other countries. Equally, they can be exposed to risks from journeys that are local (the child walking to school exposed to air pollution), or regional/national (road traffic accidents on busy motorways or freeways), or international (the risks associated with air travel). Clearly, different spatial scales of flows call forth different modes of transport (pedestrian, perhaps, or private or public transport, or by air), though access to these depends upon one's material circumstances. Similarly, the spread of disease can be local, as when a cold virus or childhood infection circulates among children in a nursery or primary school. Such spread might be contained regionally or within a national boundary. However, as we see later the porosity of such boundaries, coupled with the availability of modern air transport, means that disease spread can have a global reach.

Health-related information can be shared locally, as when a neighbour draws attention to a piece they have read in a newspaper, for example. Or it might flow within a regional or national setting, as when a regional or national health service transmits advice or information in relation to health care. But information is now carried and shared across cyberspace, such that one can glean useful (and perhaps not-so-useful) intelligence about health or medical conditions from web-sites that have originated on the other side of the world. Flows of people in order to access health care can be very local, as when short trips are taken to a primary care centre or a hospital for a consultation or treatment. Equally, they can be further afield, as when one has to travel to a regional centre for specialist treatment (for example, cancer surgery). At a yet broader spatial scale such flows can be international, as when people decide to travel abroad for medical or dental treatment (so-called 'health tourism').

It is instructive to describe the extent to which mobility has increased in *volume* over the past 50 or so years, and to outline how *modes* of travel have altered. Let me consider this in a British context. In terms of volume, the total distance travelled (other than on foot) by British people increased from 218 billon passenger kilometres in 1952, to 817 billion in 2007, a near fourfold increase (Office for National Statistics, 2010; see also Pooley et al. 2005). Pooley and his colleagues (2005: 18-33) have traced the changing transport infrastructure, which has clearly dictated changes in mode of travel. At the start of the 20th century travel between towns was primarily by train, and the network comprised some 32,000 km of track, with most areas of the country reachable by train. Since the mid 1960s this network has shrunk dramatically, with only the largest towns and cities, in the main, remaining connected. Bus and coach travel has also reduced since the early 1950s. In 1952 over 42% of trips by non-pedestrians were by coach and bus, with 27% undertaken by car. By 2007 the proportion of travel by bus and coach had shrunk to 6%, while that by car had grown to 84%, overwhelming all other forms of non-pedestrian travel within the country. Travel by bicycle in 1952 amounted to 23 billion passenger kilometres (11% of total distance travelled) but this fell to just 4 billion passenger kilometres by 2007. Pooley and his colleagues (2005: Chapter 4) describe these changes in more detail and examine differences by age group and gender. They conclude that there has been an approximate doubling of total distances travelled and in mean trip length since the mid 1960s, but little change in the *number* of trips undertaken. Knowles (2006: 411) presents further data to reveal the increase in mean distance travelled by car in the UK during the last 35 years (Table 1.1). At the same time, the mean distances travelled on foot and by bicycle have reduced, though both remain an important part of personal travel.

These data relate to a single country in the global north. Trip-making data for countries in the global south are harder to come by, a shortcoming that, in part, accounts for the anchoring of mobility studies firmly in the global north and its relative neglect in large parts of Africa and Asia (Pirie 2009a). Although a very crude indicator, data from the World Bank on the number of passenger cars per capita reveal clear contrasts between countries in the global north and south (Table 1.2). We can also point to the contrast between those who are super-mobile and the immobility of most in Africa trapped in poverty and geographical inaccessibility. Thus, rural-dwelling children in Africa may have long trips to school that inevitably diminish their possibilities for learning, while pregnant women in need of emergency obstetric care may find this completely out of reach, contributing to high rates of maternal and infant mortality (Pirie 2009a: 22). Those who migrate to African cities may find employment in city centres, but if the only affordable housing is on the periphery they will find the commuting to be lengthy, costly, and a drain on their health and well-being.

The statistics cited above are, inevitably, aggregations of vast numbers of individual trips, whether potential or actual. Many researchers have studied individual trip-making behaviour and the determinants of this and the constraints that people face. The implications of this for health and well-being are considered later.

Table 1.1   Average annual distance travelled (in miles) in the UK, by mode

Mode	1975-76	1999-2001	% change
Walking	255	189	-26
Bicycle	51	39	-24
Car	3199	5354	67
% mileage by car, van, lorry	71%	82%	
Average trip length (miles)	5.1	6.7	

Source: Knowles (2006): 411.

Table 1.2   Passenger cars per 1000 people (2007)

	'Global south'		'Global north'
Country	Cars per 1000 persons	Country	Cars per 1000 persons
Ethiopia	1	New Zealand	615
Sierra Leone	3	Germany	566
Uganda	3	France	498
Mozambique	7	UK	463
Pakistan	9	Ireland	437
Kenya	15	Canada	372
China	22	Japan	325

Source: World Bank Indicators: http://data.worldbank.org/indicator/IS.VEH.PCAR.P3 (accessed 8 October 2010).

Space-time separation

If we are to speak of movement and flow we have to understand that things move or flow from one place to another. They consume distance and cross space. I need therefore to say something about distance (spatial separation), a concept that is fundamental to geographic thought, and how such spatial separation can change over time.

Conventionally, distance is measured in physical units; formerly in 'imperial' units of yards and miles, now in metric units of metres and kilometres. But, if the pun can be forgiven, this does not get us very far. If asked how far it is from one's home to some shops, or place of work, we will often speak of the separation in terms of minutes. If asked how far from one town to another, or one city to another on a different continent, we will use hours as our measure of spatial separation, since this corresponds with our experience; we know, or can guess, what the journey times are, or are likely to be. Travel time is also socially patterned. It is perhaps faster to get from your house to your primary care physician if you have a car than if you have to make two bus journeys, with all the waiting times they entail. More dramatically, the rich businessperson in São Paulo can circumvent the city's traffic congestion by using a private helicopter to travel from the suburban home to the city centre office (Adey 2010: 96-8), thereby saving travel time.

But distance can be conceptualised in ways other than travel time. It costs money to get from one place to another, so we could measure spatial separation in terms of monetary cost. Again, unlike physical distance there is not a single 'cost distance' from one place to another. The cost of travel from Lancaster (where I live) to London depends on my mode of travel, and even within a single mode (such as rail) the cost depends on the time of day or week one travels, how far ahead any booking is made, and whether I choose to travel first or second class. Travel costs can determine whether or not there is any movement at all. If the material resources are not available, the trip is either not made, or is made with considerable hardship (as when refugees flee dangers on foot or by boat to another country).

For at least 40 years social scientists have talked about the 'death of distance' (Webber 1964, Cairncross 1997); that is, the extent to which physical proximity matters any more. If the time taken to engage in communication between Hong Kong and London is no different from that taken to communicate by telephone with a near neighbour then distance would seem to be irrelevant. If this is the case, we need to assess its implications for public health and for individuals' health experiences. There is now a wealth of interaction – virtual movement – in cyberspace, movement that involves accessing health care in new ways or becoming part of internet communities that offer support and help to many people. But while virtual travel (for shopping, social interaction, and so on) can in some cases substitute for the 'real thing' there is still sufficient material interaction to suggest that the health consequences of mobility in physical space will continue to be significant for years to come.

Associations between health and movement/interaction in cyberspace are considered later in the book. For now we can simply observe that the pace of change in information and communication technologies is such that any observations I make here are likely soon to be very dated. Having said this, some fundamental properties of cyberspace will remain important. For example, 'identity – once described as rational, stable, centred and autonomous – becomes unstable, multiple, diffuse, fluid, and manipulable because the disembodied nature of communication and relative anonymity allows you to be accepted on the basis of your words, not your appearance or accent' (Kitchin 1998: 11). The opportunities for becoming more knowledgeable about one's own health, and sharing that knowledge with others, have burgeoned, and will continue to do so, as will the possibility of purchasing treatments online. The student does not need to be co-present with her medical educator but can access learning materials online. As a practitioner, she can seek online advice from more experienced or specialist professionals, in real time, in what is known as tele-medicine and tele-healthcare (Chapter 11), areas that have now spawned their own specialist journals. Like Kitchin (1998) we can acknowledge that cyberspace confers both benefits for human health and well-being, as well as dis-benefits, features that are spelt out in more detail later.

We have seen that spatial separation can be envisaged in terms of temporal separation. Yet these travel times can themselves evolve, and have evolved as transport improvements take place. This is known as *time-space compression* or *time-space convergence*. Although sociologists and contemporary geographers have recently developed the notion of time-space compression (see Peters 2006: 52-63 for a critical account) the idea has been around for well over 40 years. In a classic paper Don Janelle (1969) introduced the concept of time-space convergence, by which he meant the ways in which innovations in transport allows places to 'approach each other' in time-space. His interest in time-space convergence was not an epidemiological one. Rather, he was concerned to show how this reduction in the friction of distance allowed for the centralisation of economic activity. My interest is how the convergence of places brings opportunities for diseases to spread more quickly.

Cliff and his colleagues (2009) illustrate time-space convergence. As they note, for most of human history 'long-distance travel, whether within countries (using streams and rivers, later canals, and coastal shipping) or between continents (using seaborne shipping), was dominantly water-dependent' (Cliff et al. 2009: 308-9). On land, until the emergence of rail travel, transport was time-consuming and often hazardous. Among the examples cited are changes in the travel times of ocean-going vessels between Europe and North America between 1820 and 1940, where travel time from London to New York reduced from 25 days in the early 19th century to 4-5 days in the late 1930s. Echoing Janelle, they sketch changes in journey time between London and Scotland, noting that by stagecoach in 1750 the journey took 11 days, reducing to 3 days by mail coach in the late 18th century and then to less than 24 hours in 1850 with the advent of the steam train. Currently, the journey time by train from London to Glasgow can be little more than 4 hours. Note the qualifier 'can be'; there is no such thing as *the* journey time between places. Much depends on mode of travel, time of day, as well as delays at the origin and destination, and on the journey itself. As a final example, consider the travel time by air from New York to California, a distance of about 3000 miles. In the 1920s this took 2 days (involving some rail travel as well) but this declined to half a day by 1960; the trip time from New York to Los Angeles is now 6 hours (less in the opposite direction). The reductions in travel time are non-linear and asymptotic; that is to say, there is a limit to the extent to which further savings in travel time are possible.

Janelle's original point was that this convergence of places is not spatially uniform. Improvements in travel mean that some places get by-passed, while others are privileged. Intermediate locations and stop-overs are, more and more, a thing of the past; at the extreme the journey times between some places *increase*, leading to time-space 'divergence'. The fact that time-distances between all pairs of places are not shrinking uniformly has clear consequences for the spread of disease. I shall have more to say about these consequences later. Suffice it to say that the closeness of Guangdong, China to Toronto in Canada is revealed in the SARS (severe acute respiratory syndrome) epidemic; 'in an epidemiological sense, "wet markets" in Guangdong, China potentially were as proximate to classrooms at York University or streetcars on Yonge Street' (Braun 2008: 259). I return briefly to SARS later in the chapter, and more fully in Chapter 9.

As Doreen Massey has argued (see Adey 2010: 91-2 and Zook and Brunn 2006), time-space convergence/compression is socially differentiated as well as geographically variable. Some social groups (such as the frequently male frequent flyers) will benefit from time-space compression, while others (such as trafficked young women from East Europe or West Africa) suffer the consequences. And many others below flight paths are not joined together at all. These inequalities should not be ignored and I seek to address them in later chapters.

Networks, network capital and globalisation

As noted earlier, geographers, cartographers and epidemiologists have, for well over 150 years, been representing health-related and medical data on maps, using geographical areas as the units of representation. These different visualisations can be incredibly powerful (see Gatrell and Elliott 2009: 49-75). But if we are interested in mobilities we have to examine and represent such flows and the networks that give rise to them. It is much less easy to visualise flows of people or goods, or diseases, than static patterns, though powerful means of visualising networks of relations are becoming available (Christakis and Fowler 2009). But what *are* such networks?

Networks are 'both objective realities that influence the patterns of disease distribution and powerful metaphors for interpreting the causes and significance of those problems' (King 2008: 210). This suggests that we need to engage with the literature on networks if we are to understand disease spread. But as I hope to show in this book, such an engagement reaps rewards beyond just the study of disease diffusion.

If we unpack the quote from King, we see that networks can be regarded as both real structures and in metaphorical terms. Both are important. For example, Richard Sennett (see Moran 2009: 179-80) reminds us of the analogies that eighteenth century urban planners drew between blood flow and urban movement. A French engineer, Pierre Patte, referred to streets as 'arteries' and 'veins' and that when urban movement slowed 'the collective body suffers a crisis of confidence like that an individual body suffers during a stroke when an artery becomes blocked'. Moran notes that the word 'arterial' was adopted in reference to British roads in the 1890s and that when the car arrived 'this medical metaphor expanded to include the idea of the traffic jam as a disease of modern life, a dysfunctional clot in the circulatory system'.

Networks are a fundamental idea in the field of social studies of science and technology ('STS') and in what has become known as *actor-network theory* (ANT). For example, in understanding disease spread we need to construct networks that are 'a hybrid of computers, communications, hospitals, health advisories, and ... medical countermeasures such as quarantine [see below] and travel restriction' (Hinchcliffe and Bingham 2008: 225). The field of the social studies of technology tells us that we cannot separate out the social from the material. Humans need objects in order to function; for example, cars and other vehicles to move, computers and iPhones to interact, and so on. Bissell (2009a) draws on these ideas in seeing the luggage accompanying the rail traveller as 'corporeal prostheses' which can both enable and encumber the traveller. The traveller is tied to her luggage which can cause 'tense thighs, sore feet and aching hands', while Bissell goes so far as to suggest (2009a: 189), perhaps somewhat exaggeratedly, that 'memories of transporting bulky or heavy objects might have the capacity to traumatise passengers'. Thus, humans and non-humans together form networks. The connections between these things matter, and are frequently examined (as in Bissell's work) in qualitative terms.

From a more quantitative perspective mathematically-minded social scientists have long been interested in the structures of social networks, structures that are formed from a set of nodes (usually people) and the social relations between them. Such social relations are frequently defined on the basis of friendship. As analytical tools and methods have developed, together with the means of handling large data sets, a literature has emerged that has begun to explore the consequences of social networks for human health and well-being. Research on how diseases spread within such networks has existed for well over 60 years and has itself been re-invigorated as the importance of networks has become more widely recognised (see Chapter 9). A very compelling recent example is work on the spread of the hospital-acquired infection, MRSA, through Dutch hospitals. Here, patients may be readmitted to several different hospitals, with university hospitals more likely to take in patients previously seen elsewhere; patients bring with them pathogens that then spread to others. 'In this way, all hospitals in the Netherlands become connected and form a network consisting of referred patients who form a bridge between hospitals and provide a path that can facilitate the spread of hospital-acquired infections, such as MRSA, between hospitals' (Donker et al. 2010). The authors construct the network of links between hospitals, showing the centrality of some – and hence their importance as nodes that speed the diffusion process.

A detailed examination of network structure and its health consequences is beyond the scope of this book, since it does not necessarily imply *mobility*. Nonetheless, it is worth brief consideration here and in doing so I draw on examples in the intriguing popular account in Christakis and Fowler (2009). As they show, networks can both promote good health, but they can also have the opposite effect. Improvements in smoking behaviour, alcohol consumption, and obesity have all been demonstrated when targeted at individuals who are centrally located in networks (and therefore in a position to influence others) rather than at randomly targeted individuals. Thus one person quitting smoking can have a positive effect on his or her friends, and friends' friends, and so on. Immunising well-connected 'hubs' in a network may be more effective than if a random sample of the population is immunised. For the authors, exploiting network structures provides 'a new foundation for public health' (Christakis and Fowler 2009: 129). However, there can be negative effects. For instance, there is strong evidence of 'suicide contagion' among teenagers, where the suicide of one person may suggest itself to other susceptible young people who have had contact with the person taking his or her life. Both boys and girls with friends who had killed themselves in the previous 12 months were 2-3 times more likely to consider suicide, and twice as likely to attempt to do so than those without such contact (Christakis and Fowler 2009: 128). The internet provides a means of developing networks in cyberspace, whereby suicide 'clubs' get established online, in countries such as Japan, for vulnerable people to collaborate in taking their lives (Rajagopal 2004).

Manuel Castells has argued that the proliferation of information and communication technologies (ICT) leads to new forms of organising social and economic life in time and space. He refers to *spaces of flows* that replace, in significance, the *space of places* in which social life is traditionally played out. For hundreds of years people were required to come together physically to exchange goods and services; now, many of these transactions can be performed remotely. We therefore have a *network society* in which instantaneous or fast flows trump conventional geographic proximity. Rosa (2003) speaks of 'social acceleration', in which social interactions get speeded up. As we shall see throughout this book, these accelerations can be both a curse and a blessing (Braun 2008: 261); for example, the networks of travel allow the rapid spread of a disease such as SARS but the communication networks among health professionals allow the rapid exchange of knowledge about a new virus.

Not everyone enjoys equal access to networks. The French sociologist Pierre Bourdieu distinguished between different forms of *capital* that accrue to people. As well as economic capital (access to monetary resources) he includes social, cultural and symbolic capital (Crossley 2005). Urry (2007) seeks to add to this set the notion of 'network capital'. (Kaufmann and Montulet 2008 prefer the term 'mobility capital', but the idea is the same). It refers to 'the real and potential *social relations* that mobilities afford' (Urry 2007: 196, my emphasis). It is the ability or capacity to form and maintain social relations with people who are not co-present, thereby adding financial, cultural and (perhaps) emotional benefit. Those people rich in network capital are those with access to numerous resources for interaction; such resources including material objects (money, technologies, communication devices, documents), other people, and time. Urry contrasts network capital with social capital, as theorised by the American sociologist Robert Putnam (2000). This too is *relational*, in the sense that it emerges as a result of social relations among individuals in communities. But Urry criticises Putnam for over-emphasising the importance of spatial proximity – the tight-knit local communities that have attracted the interest of politicians and policy-makers. Urry prefers to stress 'at-a-distance' relationships as much as those based on propinquity.

As with other forms of capital, network capital is unevenly distributed, whether by age, class, income, race, gender or disability. Not all people are mobile. Not all people wish to be mobile. Some people are constrained by physical impairments, others by economic circumstances. For example, the woman in a one-car household, working at home and looking after two pre-school children is less mobile than her partner who works away from home (with his car) during the week. And among those who do move, vast numbers do so under duress, hardship or as a result of conflict and war. To some extent the mobilities turn led by sociologists has, surprisingly, neglected this. In establishing a new mobilities paradigm it has not always been acknowledged that access to network capital is unevenly distributed and socially patterned. Fifty years ago, and more, human mobility in the developed world was constrained by the friction of distance; it remains so for many social groups. In the global south the constraints of distance remain considerable because of poor transport infrastructure, even if the new mobile communications technologies are penetrating new markets in resource-poor countries.

Mobility, then, is socially patterned, even hierarchically organised. Cresswell (2006) draws an important distinction between the kinetic elite (those occupying prime locations in social space, the possessors of large stocks of network capital) and the kinetic underclass, those who move less freely. Citing Zygmunt Bauman, he suggests that globalization 'is tied to the dreams and desires of the kinetic elite who inhabit the luxurious space of flows, and who need the kinetic underclass to service it. There are no *tourists* without *vagabonds*' (Cresswell 2006: 256, his italics).

The vagrant, the vagabond, the hobo, the asylum seeker are the 'othered' mobile, those at the margins of mobile society; some of these others may choose the mobile life, but many do not. But whether they do so or not they are at the bottom of the social pile, with few prospects of upwards mobility in social space. They often create anxiety among those who are more fortunate. As Cresswell (1997) has demonstrated, those who are 'out of place' because of their mobility are often imbued with metaphorical constructions of disease or infection. Such metaphors 'mobilize different ways of dealing with displacement, but the end is the same – to restore things to their *proper place*' (Cresswell 1997: 342, his italics).

We should expect – even demand – that those working in public health have inequalities at the forefront of their agendas. In the context of human movement there are some writers who certainly do. Paul Farmer (2005) speaks of the 'pathologies of power that transcend all borders'. Clarence Tam (2006) has considered the health of human migrants, not in the narrow sense of how healthy they are in comparison with non-movers (see some of the discussion in Chapter 7) but in terms of their positioning within the context of global and regional, political and economic, regimes. With specific reference to those on the US-Mexican border he suggests that many migrants from Mexico are subject to 'structural violence', by which he means less the physical brutalities (though these take place) and more the lack of human rights, and the poor wages, that such people endure. The same violence is done to those women moving overseas as domestic workers. As Anbesse and colleagues (2009) reveal in their study of Ethiopian domestic workers in the Middle East women may be subject to all kinds of exploitation and *restricted* movement. At one level (or scale – the international) they are clearly mobile but once relocated they encounter mobility constraints. They have relocated spatially but are dislocated socially. They are at once mobile and immobile. Where social networks among women from the same cultural group are established, and not disrupted by employers, these help such women maintain their mental health and well-being and to show resilience in the face of adversity.

As Tam puts it 'public health should not merely constitute the maintenance of a state of "absence of disease", but should be a pro-active enterprise striving for equity and social justice, with human rights at its core and "health" as the main intended outcome of such activity' (Tam 2006: 4). But he also acknowledges that since health services are provided by nation states, with an emphasis on their own populations, it is difficult to meet the needs of mobile populations. Public health has to transcend borders and be shaped less by the state and corporations and more by the needs of the disenfranchised (Tam 2006: 5).

Networks evolve, get re-structured, and can be disrupted. We shall see examples of this later in the book, but for now consider how movement gets disrupted by natural hazards, such as flooding, earthquakes or tsunamis. If bridges get destroyed, and roads so badly damaged that they become impassable, then normal patterns of spatial behaviour have to change. Trips may become impossible, or at least seriously altered, as alternative routes have to be negotiated. What might have been a 10 minute journey to a doctor could become a two hour journey, as happened in West Cumbria, England, in January 2010 after major flooding. Many readers will recall the major disruptions to tens of thousands of people (and businesses and other organisations) following the release of ash from the eruption of the Icelandic volcano, Eyjafjallajökull, in April 2010. The suspension of flights clearly had some environmental (and possibly health) benefits (see Chapter 4) but caused enormous stress to those who suffered the expense and inconvenience of delayed journeys. A special issue of the journal *Mobilities* (2011 Vol. 6, No. 1) has explored the impact of the eruption on human mobility.

As noted earlier, if we wish to understand networked flows of people, information, disease and healthcare, we need to do so at a variety of spatial scales, from the global to the local. We might argue that, of these scales, the global is absolutely critical. I need therefore to say something about *globalization*. This is a process of greater integration within the world economy, realised by movements of goods and services, capital, and labour, leading to economic decisions being shaped by global conditions. It involves: increasing inter-connectivity among places, particularly among major world cities; increasing speed of flows between such places; and the potential both for global events to have local impacts and also events at a local scale having an impact that is global in reach. Crucially, as far as this book is concerned, it involves increasing amounts of long-distance travel to places.

As we shall see in later chapters, particularly in relation to recent and contemporary disease spread, this latter aspect is especially relevant. The point is made neatly in an editorial (29 March 2003) in Toronto's *Globe and Mail*, with respect to the spread of SARS to Canada: 'Globalization means that if someone in

China sneezes, someone in Toronto may one day catch a cold. Or something worse – if, in Guangdong province, 80 million people live cheek by jowl with chickens, pigs and ducks, so, in effect, do we all. Global village indeed' (cited in van Wagner 2008: 13). In another discussion of SARS Keil and Ali (2008b: 165) suggest that globalisation has created a network of global cities 'not joined through unilateral and unidirectional hierarchical links but through topological, multi-relational, and constitutive relationships that are performed through the bodies of migrants as much as through the socio-technical networks that sustain them'. What, then, is this network of global cities?

Peter Taylor and his research group on Global World Cities at Loughborough University have been at the forefront of research into the formation and operation of a global or world city network (see Taylor 2004, and Zook and Brunn 2006). Following Castells, he sees cities less as places and more in terms of their organisation into a network of relations. Global cities may be defined as 'key points in the organization of the global economy, and increasingly derive their functional importance from their mutual interactions rather than with their proper hinterlands' (Derudder et al. 2008: 6). As Taylor reminds us, the notion of cities formed into networks is not a feature solely of late modernity; cities were organised as regional systems during the middle ages. However, the advent of modern transport systems, and (tele)communications and information technologies, coupled with the functions of finance and services performed in cities, has given rise to a contemporary concern with describing and analysing the structure and function of a global city network.

What data are available on the flows of money, services and people between these global cities? For obvious reasons of commercial confidentiality there are few sources on the first two sets of flows. Derudder and his colleagues (2005, 2008) have reviewed sources of data on air passenger flows that can be used to inform global city network research. But they point to a number of problems with available data sets. For example, most existing data tables show stop-overs rather than the trip as a whole. As a result, less important cities appear as significant nodes simply because they are transfer points or hubs (for example, Frankfurt, or Amsterdam) on the airline network. A further problem is that data tend to represent international flows rather than flows between major cities; thus major flows between New York and Los Angeles, for example, get downplayed. Also, existing data cannot readily distinguish business from tourist flows. This matters for researchers who are interested more in the former than the latter; it matters less to those of us interested in how movement facilitates disease transmission, since a virus does not care too much whether the body belongs to a 50 year old business person or a young child.

Derudder and his colleagues use the Marketing Information Data Transfer database, containing data (for 2001) on over 500 million passenger movements, to construct an origin-destination matrix for over 300 cities, and then analyse the most significant flows or links. However, this seems to privilege several within-country flows (for example, the fourth-sixth highest volume flows are between,

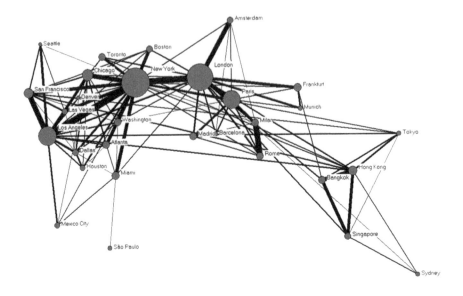

**Figure 1.1   Most important global air links according to Marketing
               Information Data Transfer (MIDT), 2001**

Source: Derudder and Witlox (2005). Reprinted with permission.

respectively: Melbourne-Sydney; Milan-Rome; and Cape Town-Johannesburg.
Nonetheless, if the 30 most important cities in terms of total volume of passengers
are considered, the flows between them reveal an interesting spatial structure
(Figure 1.1), though one that omits mainland China, India, Africa, and South
America!

    Why are such global flows and structures of relevance to the study of health?
The answer is put very neatly by Elbe (2008: 117): 'the very attempt to create a
world economy in which goods and people traverse the planet with growing ease
and speed increases the chances of pathological viruses doing exactly the same
– and with potentially devastating international social, economic and political
consequences'.

Risk and exposure

I referred earlier to the 'risk society'. Some commentators have re-defined risk as
the 'new normal', a 'state of accepted economic and personal insecurity driven by
the demands of the global marketplace' (Hooker 2006: 192). The phrase seems to
have appeared after the terrorist attacks on the World Trade Center in New York
City on September 11th 2001 but has become particularly apposite during the
banking-led economic crisis that started in 2007. Hooker suggests that the healthy
citizen of the 'new normal' is, in part, someone who is vigilant to risk and prepared

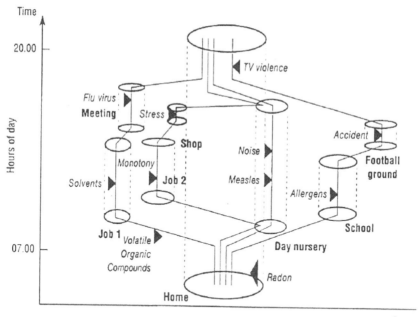

Figure 1.2   The time geography of an imaginary Swedish family

Source: Gatrell and Elliott (2009), original due to Anders Schaerstrom.

for the unexpected. Writers on health (and particularly on SARS) bracket disease and (in)security, as I show in the following section.

I want here want to say more about the encountering of risks while on the move and how this might be conceptualised in terms of time-space budgets. In particular, we can conceive of people being at risk, or exposed to various threats and environmental stressors, in different places or via different modes of travel (Curtis 2010). Geographers and epidemiologists have sought to excavate such risks, and we can do so in terms of the trajectories people trace out in time-space.

The original work on time geography was undertaken by the Swedish geographer Torsten Hägerstrand in the 1960s, and a simple hypothetical example (due to Anders Schaerstrom) suggests its relevance to health geographies (Figure 1.2). Here, we consider four members of an imaginary family, with the male partner leaving home and travelling in his car (perhaps being exposed to volatile organic compounds in his car journey) and working in a factory that might expose him to solvents or (when in meetings) to circulating viruses. His female partner takes a pre-school child to nursery (where, again, viruses may be circulating) while she herself works in a monotonous job (perhaps in an office) before encountering the stresses of shopping and commuting home. This is of course entirely hypothetical; nonetheless, it is suggestive of the fact that, in various settings and in various *journeys*, people are exposed to things that affect their health and well-being (see another schematic example in Meade and Emch 2010: 204-6). Moreover, in tracing space-time paths, the approach indicates how these paths cross, in the form of joint or shared activities; the social relations can be directly visualised. Further, it is suggestive of the constraints that people face; we cannot be in different places at the same time, and certain groups (the low paid, women juggling employment and child care) have their mobility behaviour more constrained than others.

Mei-Po Kwan has been at the forefront of attempts to explore these issues empirically, drawing upon geo-referenced data and activity diaries to map the complexity of space-time paths in urban environments. Taking data on almost 4500 households (over 10,000 individuals) in Portland, Oregon, she mapped their activity and travel patterns over a two-day period (involving almost 130,000 activities and over 71,000 trips) using sophisticated interactive spatial analytic tools within a Geographic Information Systems (GIS) framework (Kwan and Lee 2004). These paths vary with age and gender, with both young children and older adults (depending on personal circumstances – such as family income and levels of disability) having more restricted ranges of movement. More recently (Ren and Kwan 2007), she has sought to analyse and represent such paths both in physical space and cyberspace. Cyberspatial interactions are, of course, not constrained by geographical space. Kwan uses data on numbers and types of websites visited, the duration of time spent on particular sites, and connection speeds, to produce space-time paths that are 'hybrid', in the sense of tracing routes in both physical space and cyberspace. The hypothetical example shown in Figure 1.2 proves inadequate, as it is grounded in geographical space (Miller 2004; Couclelis 2009). It presupposes that activities take place at fixed locations and that any mobility is a geographical movement. But in cyberspace there is no longer a simple mapping of activities onto locations, as 'people can shop from their home or workplace, carry on business transactions from their car, socialize while walking down the street, engage in high-tech forms of entertainment while sitting in a classroom, or work for a living while sipping cappuccinos at the corner café' (Couclelis 2009: 1559). Observable trajectories in space remain paramount but we need to trace such trajectories in cyberspace too.

How does this link to health? As the hypothetical example in Figure 1.2 suggests, in occupying discrete locations, and in moving from place to place, people are exposed to risks of various kinds. Of course, in advanced economies these risks may be serious and insidious, though they pale into insignificance compared with those faced by some in the global south. The use of new location-aware, portable or wearable, technologies can help track movements (Rainham et al. 2010). Vazquez-Prokopec and colleagues (2008) have explored the use of Global Positioning Systems (GPS) data-loggers to track the movements of individuals potentially exposed to dengue fever in Peru. As the cost, quality of batteries, size and wearability of these devices improve we should – subject to appropriate ethical safeguards – see an increased use of these technologies in monitoring human movement and relating this to real exposure to infections or environmental contamination. In Chapter 3, I show how personal exposure monitoring is of use in looking at associations between respiratory disease and air quality while traversing urban environments and heavily-trafficked streets.

It would be wrong to suggest that mobility is risky business. Of course it is in some contexts. Yet in plenty of other contexts, as we see in the next chapters, mobility can add to our well-being, either because the journey itself is pleasurable or we anticipate what lies at the journey's end. Journeys can induce nostalgia just as much as places do. Equally, the virtual connections we make in cyberspace can be fruitful as well as threatening. Networks can be sustaining and create and maintain resilience; they are not only structures that aid the spread of disease.

Spatial diffusion, borders, and bio-security

Spatial diffusion refers to the spread of ideas, information, objects and diseases across geographic space and is a fundamental concept in human geography. My interest here is in the spread of infectious disease – the paths such infections take, the rates of spread and the possibilities for controlling such spread. Clearly, disease spread depends upon the means of transport and, as noted already (and expanded upon in Part 3) historically such spread was heavily constrained by geographic distance but more recently has been speeded up by international air travel.

Traditionally, geographers distinguished between 'contagious' and 'hierarchical' diffusion. The former was so-called because it relies on direct contact and is a process strongly influenced by distance because nearby places and people have a much higher probability of contact than those further away. Hierarchical diffusion refers to spread down an urban or regional hierarchy, with a disease perhaps having its origin in a major urban centre, then leapfrogging geographic space (via a transport network) to reach smaller towns and subsequently villages and small settlements. To some extent the nomenclature is unfortunate, since there has to be some form of contact in both cases – the only difference is that one is constrained by geographic distance and the other by relative location in an urban or regional hierarchy. In general, we may speak of infectious or transmissible diseases that require a susceptible person (sometimes abbreviated to a 'susceptible') to come into contact with an infectious person (an 'infective') or be exposed to environments that have been contaminated by infectives. Other infectious diseases are transmitted via vectors such as insects. In all these cases mobilities, including the movement of people and material objects, are of fundamental importance, for if infectives are able to move relatively freely the possibilities for disease transmission are greatly enhanced.

Aside from distance or relative location, what are some of the constraints to such flow – the kinds of physical barriers that are in place, or are *deliberately* put in place, to impede disease spread? These can include restrictions on the flow of people and goods, as a means of controlling the spread of infections. How are state borders policed and how permeable do they remain? How are networks managed?

Drawing on Foucault and others, Hinchcliffe and Bingham (2008) consider the management of 'biosecurity' – the risks engendered by the flows of pathogens such as viruses (and not merely, in a narrow sense, protection against bio-terrorism: see also Fidler 2006). These concern managing, first, the security of the nation-state and the securing of territory and the policing of borders; second, the security of the population, in particular securing its health and well-being; and, third, the security of 'vital systems', securing both the state and its population from technological and environmental hazards. Security in this context, then, moves beyond the defence of borders from armed aggressors and the maintenance of border integrity towards dealing with the less visible threat of viruses. Maintaining (bio)security demands surveillance, policing, regulation and control. Nation states have for many years established the machinery (visas, for example) necessary to control crossing the national frontier. Ingram (2008) uses the term 'domopolitics' to describe this privileging of the domestic (hence, 'domo') arena over the foreign body, particularly bodies that are uninvited and illegal. In many cases, and for many people, the border crossings are quite permeable, and the only issue is the tedium of queuing for the passport to be inspected. For others, and in different contexts, the experience is very different: one of rigorous scrutiny and search, harassment, and perhaps confinement. For them, international travel is only ever stressful.

Warren and his colleagues (2010) have also addressed issues of bio-security, particularly with reference to the 'swine flu' (H1N1) pandemic in 2009 (see also Chapter 9). As they note, the discourse draws on conventional security studies that sees the 'inside' as safe and secure and the 'outside' as threatening and dangerous; the threat in bio-security studies coming from infectious disease. Containment is virtually impossible, not least because of the growth in air traffic; as the authors note, in 1968 (the date of the last major influenza pandemic) there were some 261 million air travellers, but this had grown almost ten-fold to more than 2 billion in 2008. Further, the rate of spread has speeded up. Attention has shifted to the airport as a site for control, or to states (such as China) which were monitoring airline passengers waiting to disembark. They report a newspaper article in the UK. 'Quarantine officers, dressed in surgical masks, gloves and medical suits, greet passengers once the plane has docked and file silently down the aisles, placing a temperature gun at the forehead of each passenger. Anyone with a temperature even slightly above normal is singled out, removed from the plane and taken to hospital by ambulance for further tests' (from Warren et al. 2010: 732). Set against this dramatisation, others (Shu et al. 2005) claim that fever screening at airports (in Taiwan) is undoubtedly effective; using dengue fever as an example, they suggest that airport screening substantially reduces the time taken to diagnose the disease, thus being both an effective form of surveillance and preventing costly spread within the country.

The role of the World Health Organization (WHO) in policing the spread of infectious disease has been examined by Davies (2008). Her argument is that the surveillance and control exercised by WHO (or, at least, its attempts to exercise control over disease spread across borders) privileges worries in the west (or global north) over the prevention of disease outbreaks at source. The threat of disease only becomes such, she argues, when it is the *west* that feels threatened. WHO has developed a Global Outbreak and Alert Response Network (GOARN) that seeks to detect and manage outbreaks but sees such containment as the main response and its primary responsibility, rather than looking 'upstream' at the structural determinants of disease outbreaks. GOARN relies on the cooperation of nation states to help verify and manage an outbreak, cooperation that might be reluctantly given if such countries are then going to be demonised as lacking bio-security (and suffering the economic consequences). Another system, GPHIN (the Global Public Health Intelligence Network, based in Canada) monitors online news information rather than case reports: see Weir and Mykhalovskiy (2006). Like GOARN, this by-passes individual states but does provide the basis for local intervention and control. Davies argues that western countries are pleased to have a 'non-state actor' such as the WHO acting on their behalf to safeguard their borders from microbial traffic. The WHO has, in turn, seen its stature grow in recent years as it has dealt with new diseases such as SARS.

While vaccination, in order to create immunity in susceptible populations, remains one form of control it is of more interest in the present context to consider control mechanisms that seek to block mobility. These spatial strategies are designed to prevent the mixing of infectives and susceptibles, and this is done using *quarantine*. The term derives from the period of time – 40 ('quaranta') days – that was deemed appropriate in 15th century Italian states for an infection to have run its course.

A quarantine ring (sometimes called 'cordon sanitaire') is used in two ways. In 'defensive isolation' a spatial barrier is placed around an area infected with the disease, as a way of containing the disease by preventing infected individuals from 'escaping' to infect those without the disease. In 'offensive containment' barriers are placed around an uninfected area to prevent those with the disease gaining access. Andrew Cliff and his colleagues (2009) describe in detail the considerable lengths to which Italian republics and principalities went, over many years, to protect themselves from plague. Gensini et al. (2004) consider that isolation should refer to the separation and confinement of known infectives, while quarantine is a term that should be restricted to suspected carriers of a disease.

As Cliff and colleagues note, the use of these spatial strategies may have been appropriate in a pre-modern era of slow maritime travel. It is far from clear how they might work in a modern and late-modern era of rapid transport, when the travel time from *a* to *b* is substantially less than the incubation period of an infection. It is also far from clear just what scope nation-states have, in the 21st century, to control such spread and just how effective international agencies such as WHO can be. On the latter, Elbe (2008: 123) notes that the need 'to coordinate responses with a large number of member states places serious constraints on the speed in which international organizations can mount an effective response to any new virus'. There have often been tensions between governments who regard their nation-state as wholly autonomous and the roles that supra-national organisations feel they could and should play in managing global risks. For example, China attempted initially to suppress news of the SARS outbreak but internet and other communications traffic rendered this impossible. Subsequently China acknowledged the outbreak and WHO re-asserted its role as an international organisation.

Regardless of the relative roles played by nation-states and international organisations, the securitisation of disease risk has not gone uncriticised. This is because it tends to focus on ways of detecting outbreaks and managing disease spread rather than dealing with the causes of the disease in the first place. A good example would be the emphasis given to transmission of HIV which, like SARS and pandemic influenza, has long been regarded as a threat to international peace and security (see Ingram 2008 for a discussion of this). Clearly, we need a good understanding of how this disease, and others, spreads (and I consider this later). But now we have such an understanding it would be more valuable to focus attention and resources on the structural factors (of which poverty and global inequalities are the prime candidates: see Farmer 2005) that are the primary drivers of HIV and other infections. As Elbe (2008) notes, we need less attention to the military metaphors (of 'threat' and 'battle') and the securitisation of viruses, and more to the structural political and economic factors that constrain an effective international response. Fidler (2006: 208-9) has made much the same remarks about the US BioWatch program, where sensors designed to detect bio-weapons agents have been placed in American cities. This initiative illustrates how bio-security policy in the United States focuses on national interests rather than broader global needs.

Concluding remarks

If there is an over-arching theme in the present book it is that mobilities can affect our health and well-being (and vice-versa). Sometimes they can promote good health and offer opportunities for healthcare. But at other times mobilities can impact adversely on our health and well-being. It is a mapping of these different effects and relationships that I attempt in what follows. My attention is focused on sets of things that move in geographical space, whether locally, regionally or globally, or in cyberspace, and the consequences that such flows have for human health and healthcare. Having in this chapter outlined some concepts to help inform subsequent discussion, I begin the 'journey' (if you will) by looking at the links between physical movement – slow and fast travel – and human health and well-being.

Part 1: Travel

In this first part of the book I consider both how our experience of the world using different modes of travel serves to maintain or add to our sense of well-being and, conversely, how these different travel modes may impact negatively on human health. Travel can do us good, but it can engender risk.

Unlike much of the recently emerging mobilities literature I am not especially concerned with mobility as a social and cultural engagement; I *am* interested in whether the journey itself is a means of deriving pleasure or benefit to mental health and well-being. As the urban planner Kevin Lynch pointed out many years ago: 'We might think of travel as a pleasure, rather than a brief and necessary evil...Any comparative measurement of access must account for the benefits of moving, as well as just arriving' (cited in Jensen 2009: xvi). Ingold (2007) distinguishes between 'transport' as goal-directed or oriented towards the destination, and 'wayfaring' as an active engagement with the journey itself. As Aitchison and her colleagues (2000: 29) note in their review of literature on leisure and tourism landscapes, while considerable attention has been paid to such landscapes relatively little attention has been given 'to the appreciation of scenes observed *en route* to the destination...[T]he journey can be regarded not simply as a means to an end but as a source of pleasure derived from a sense of freedom through travel'.

There is a wealth of mobilities literature on *forms* of travel – ethnographic studies of the uses of cars and planes, and the associated material infrastructures. One writer on automobile driving suggests that it 'can be decomposed into multiple accountable, locally identifiable and morally charged actions...which require their reflexive use in relation to time-bound spaces to maintain the endogenous production of motorway traffic' (Laurier 2004: 270). Here I concentrate, much more prosaically, on the health gains, but also the dis-benefits, resulting from such travel. Much of the mobilities literature in cultural studies and social science relates to commonly-used modes of travel (with most attention given to automobiles and airplanes), but there is interesting research to be undertaken on the impacts on well-being of more mundane forms of travel (by boat, bus, and rail, for example: see the collection edited by Vannini 2009, a set of interesting ethnographic essays that do not have anything directly to say about health and well-being). The much-studied 'hypermobility' represented by air travel and globalised networks needs to give way to an examination of 'routes less travelled' (Vannini 2009: 10). I seek to do so in what follows.

The conventional view in transport planning is that travel is a disutility to be minimized (Mokhtarian 2005: 93) and, for the business traveller, a cost to the employer (Lyons and Urry 2005). Yet, as Mokhtarian's title suggests, travel can be a desired end in itself, not merely an instrumental means of getting from one place to another. It can satisfy a need for: adventure; new environmental experiences; control; variety; escape; and physical exercise. All these needs – not simply the last, most obvious one – are related to health and well-being. The liking for travel (Ory and Mokhtarian 2005) extends to routine urban travel, not only the vacation trip, and for different modes of travel too. Ory and Mokhtarian find (in a survey of commuters in the San Francisco Bay Area) that the daily commute is enjoyed by one-fifth of their sample (albeit that a third dislike it), though well over one half of their sample like or very much like social or entertainment-related trips. It is difficult to separate out the influence of the prospective destination in shaping the desirability or otherwise of the trip.

Clearly, travel time need not be unproductive and there are useful and positive activities that can be undertaken, depending on the mode of travel. Plenty of commentators and researchers are arguing in favour of slowness and a reversal of the 'logic of acceleration'. In an interesting essay, Pallasmaa (2008: 152) suggests that 'a distinct slowness reveals the depth and detail of life, whereas speed and mobility wipe those dimensions away, causing a sense of intolerable flatness, sameness and boredom' (see also Bergmann 2008a, in the same volume). Peters (2006: 42) makes the same point: 'by introducing slower cars, more bicycles, more walking, the world will return to a more restful state', conferring health benefits on both individuals and wider society.

Considerable attention has been, and continues to be, paid to walking, cycling, car and air travel as part of the fabric of late-modern society. But, as noted in Chapter 1, the mobilities literature has little to say about health, certainly the negative environmental and health impacts of mass car ownership. In the first three chapters I want to ensure that the risks, dangers, exposures to pollution, and so on, are excavated. As I shall show, these dis-benefits impact both on the users of transport and also on others close by.

In the final chapter in this first part of the book I consider travel not according to mode but, rather, purpose. Specifically, I want to explore some of the connections between tourism and health. We go on vacation to 'recharge our batteries'; so to what extent does the vacation allow us to do so? Yet, as with different modes of transport, vacations and tourism can bring dis-benefits. Thus I examine some of the epidemiological literature on the risk of excess exposure to the sun. Last, I consider the consequences of travelling for the specific purpose of engaging in sexual activity. What are the health impacts of this, both for the tourist and host populations?

Chapter 2
Walking and Cycling

Introduction

I need first to re-assert that walking and cycling are forms of transport; they move people from one place to another. While this may seem obvious, especially to those with a public health imagination, it is often the case that motorised transport is privileged and that cycling and walking are merely seen as leisure activities or as exercise that has to be promoted for the public good (Woodcock and Aldred 2008). To some extent too, the speeding up of social life or what Freund and Martin (2004: 277) refer to as the 'time squeeze' puts pressure on us to get things done quickly and to minimise travel time; this leads to the 'disappearance of that musing, unstructured space in which so much thinking, courting, daydreaming, and seeing has transpired' (Solnit, quoted in Freund and Martin 2004: 277). For those leading hectic lives walking and cycling in natural settings are replaced by the treadmill or cycling machine, either at home or the gym; mobility of a sort perhaps, but a rather poor substitute for the real thing and a cultural form that commodifies non-motorised transport and which segregates the user from the web of everyday life (Freund and Martin 2004: 280).

As Urry (2007) observes, there are many ways to walk; walking can be relatively mundane (such as a walk to a local shop or store), a means to fulfilment (such as climbing a hill) or, at an extreme, a forced march (Urry 2007: 65). In the developed world walking can be a pleasurable outdoor activity, particularly where the aim is to enjoy the landscape and the walk itself. Walking and cycling may generate health gains from maintaining a fit body. In resource-poor countries walking may be a necessity (to fetch food, water, or firewood) or a means of escaping persecution during times of war and conflict (see Chapter 6). We do well to remind ourselves (Aitchson et al. 2000: 29) that the old spelling of 'travaile' calls to mind the link between mobility (travel), hard work and physical discomfort (travail).

The chapter is organised into four sections. I first consider walking for leisure, before, second, turning attention to the gains people can reap for physical health and, third, to cycling, with the sub-title taken from a famous quote by a former British Conservative politician who cajoled those made unemployed by his government's policies to 'get on your bike' to look for work. The final section explores the exposures of walkers and cyclists to air pollution.

Rambling and strolling

Urry (2007: 36-8) and Peters (2006: 28-36) point to some of the pleasures involved in pedestrian travel. These may be relatively simple ones of meeting up with friends, relatives and colleagues in various settings. But other pleasures lie in the experience of travel itself, including the sights and settings encountered and enjoyed on the way. Urry reminds us of the travels on foot enjoyed daily by the Lake District poets in the early 19th century, whereby walking became a way of being, not simply a means of travel (Urry 2007: 79). Walking tours served to connect the person to the landscape as well as providing private emotional sustenance and refreshment of body and soul. In the first half of the 20th century 'cycling and hiking revolved around the notion of "open air" thought to make people better, as they experience open, panoramic, uninhibited scenery and very lengthy walks' (Urry 2007: 81). Walks were less a slow amble and more an active ramble.

Most of us – certainly among the able-bodied – can attest to the enjoyment of walking, whether along a beach, in the hills, or among an interesting urban area. Walking is therapeutic, a means of (re)connecting with nature, and the 'therapy' may lie either in the solitary walk or in the company of others, whether during day-time or at night. But, of course, context is everything; if the beach is polluted or crowded, the hills have poorly maintained footpaths, and the urban areas are perceived to be dangerous or dull, the walk may be more health-damaging than health-promoting.

Nineteenth-century London and Paris saw young, single men 'walking without a definite route, distracted and concerned with adventure, entertainment and sexual pleasure' – a kind of 'promiscuous ramble' (Urry 2007: 67). In Paris the male ramblers were known as flâneurs. Note the distinctively male occupation, and the invisible female; as in some contemporary cities, the ramble was not without risk to women of any age who might find themselves harassed by unwelcome male attention and perhaps suffer the consequences. Walking unaccompanied during the day, but among many strangers in a busy street, may be perfectly safe, in contrast to a night-time journey through poorly-lit and quite deserted streets. It is interesting to observe how British town centres change their character during the day; filled with couples and family groups enjoying shopping and strolls in the afternoon, they can appear much more threatening in the evenings when groups of young (and middle-aged) men and women arrive on the scene to 'party'. Equally, an urban environment where there is a lot to see and enjoy is likely to be more conducive to well-being than a walk through an uninteresting housing estate that, if not entirely lifeless, may be sparsely populated with people perceived (rightly or wrongly) to be threatening as a result of their behaviour or appearance.

In rural areas, leisure walking is a relatively new phenomenon. Before the nineteenth century walking was seen as a sign of poverty and even madness, while landscapes now seen as iconic (the English Lake District, the European Alps) were previously regarded as inhospitable and perhaps dangerous. The solitary traveller was regarded with suspicion. As the Romantic movement took hold the mountains and hills were considered worth walking and exploring – places to rejuvenate the senses. Between the two World Wars there developed new enthusiasms for rambling and hiking, activities engaged in by groups of people less for relaxation and more for strengthening body and soul, particularly when the weather was inclement (Urry 2007: 81); the countryside was seen as energising. But while fresh air and exercise was provided in the nineteenth and twentieth centuries for factory workers who could escape the cities to traverse extensive networks of footpaths, landowners did their best to restrict access (Aitchison et al. 2000: 55-58). Despite these barriers, by the early 1930s there were half a million regular walkers in the countryside.

This activity led to the formation of the Ramblers' Association in the UK (now simply 'Ramblers'), a charity whose origins lay in the wish to provide better access to open spaces for walkers. Formally speaking the organisation was established in 1930, but groups were formed in the nineteenth century to protect access to footpaths, and the first federation of groups of ramblers took place in Glasgow, with the formation of the West of Scotland Ramblers' Alliance in 1892. Before this, a number of walking clubs had been set up in and near London, including the Sunday Tramps in 1879 and the Forest Ramblers Club in 1884 (see: www.ramblers.org.uk/aboutus/history). The Ramblers Association started with 1200 members and campaigned for the establishment of a network of long distance paths. In the twentieth century the middle classes discovered rambling 'as an activity to promote good health and companionship, demonstrating its attraction as a sociable as well as a solitary activity' (Aitchison et al. 2000: 57). Vigorous long-distance walking could be combined with the enjoyment of natural surroundings and conversation with others.

In 2010 there were over 140,000 members who support the charity's aims 'to promote walking for health, leisure and transport to everyone, of all ages, backgrounds and abilities, in towns and cities as well as in the countryside'. Such promotion depends on the motivation of individuals and their willingness to participate in the activity either alone or in the company of others; but it also depends on knowing where to walk. The Ramblers now issue new members with automatic computer links to their nearest group and have mobilised social networking sites to put members in touch with each other.

Wylie (2005) has described in great detail the experience of a solitary day's walk along a coastal path in south-west England. His aim is to present the walk 'as a mosaic of moods, incidents, introspections, speculations about landscapes and bodies' (Wylie 2005: 237). Drawing upon a range of post-structuralist thinking, and citing Derrida, he claims that a walker 'is poised between the country ahead and the country behind, between one step and the next...between there and not-there, perpetually caught in an apparitional process of arriving/departing' (p. 237). As he admits, pressing 'perhaps tortuous theoretical propositions into service on behalf of a walk by the sea, along cliffs, and through fields may seem quixotic' (236-7). More prosaically, he acknowledges the pain (feet, knees, hips) of a long walk and this has to be set against the emotional benefits which Wylie hints at. Others are quite clear about these benefits. For example, the poet Simon Armitage writes that 'there's a sense of creativity about it, and a sense of wellbeing that you are getting the organs and the lungs and the blood moving. You never come back from a walk feeling worse'. Another British poet, the appropriately named Andrew Motion, suggests that 'the rhythm of walking and rhythm of writing and poetry are very easily combined...the movement of the body releases a poem and then confirms its rhythmic identity...walking gives you ideas, unblocks blockages, sets up rhythms in your head' (interviews in the *Guardian* newspaper, 17 November 2010).

At an extreme, for some it is the real physical bodily effort that provides motivation, and only if this is experienced is the walk (or, more usually, climb) judged 'worth it'. In Scotland, Sir Charles Munro challenged people to climb all the mountain peaks higher than 3000 feet (283 in total) and 'bagging' the Munros remains an activity striven for by many.

Walking for health

Let me now say something about more purposive walking, beginning with a discussion of walking as a means of securing child health.

The proportion of children walking to school in Britain has changed greatly in the last 20 years (Office for National Statistics, 2010). In 1990 62% of children aged 5-10 years walked to school, but this had fallen to 48% by 2008; there was also a decline among 11-16 year olds (from 48% to 40%). However, in an important book, Pooley and his colleagues (2005) suggest that the walk to school continues to be a very important aspect of mobility that has changed little in significance over the past 60 years. What are the consequences of walking for the health of young people, and what initiatives are appropriate to ensure that it promotes good health, rather than having negative effects?

Many schools, supported by government and health authorities, encourage active commuting, not least as a means of addressing serious contemporary problems of obesity in the developed world. Obesity has become a major source of public health concern – even panic – in the west, and the literature on this, and on how to address it, has mushroomed in the last few years. What is the scale of the problem? In 2001 it was reported that 8.5% of 6 year olds and 15% of 15 year olds in the UK were obese (Mackett et al. 2005), though more recent data from the National Childhood Measurement Programme (2009-10) indicate that almost a quarter of English children starting school, and one-third of those leaving primary school, were overweight or obese (www.ic.nhs.uk/ncmp).

The therapeutic benefits of children walking (or engaging in other physical activity, such as cycling, swimming, organised sport, and dance) have long been recognised. Evidence suggests that physical fitness during early adolescence confers health benefits (improved cardiovascular health) in adulthood (Timperio et al. 2004). Indeed, walking has been described as 'near perfect exercise' (Ogilvie et al. 2007). It is generally convenient, straightforward (at least, for those without physical impairments), popular, carbon-neutral, and appropriate for all ages. Mackett and his colleagues (2005) studied nearly 200 children aged 10-13 years in Hertfordshire, UK and found that walking is almost as effective as structured ball games in consuming calories; as a free activity, requiring no preparation or equipment, it is an attractive intervention as far as public health policy is concerned. More recently, Cooper and colleagues (2010) found that physical activity (measured using accelerometers) is 43% higher among children walking to school than for those travelling by car; further, it exceeds that in the playground. What these papers do not address is the quality of the walk, including exposure to traffic volume and pollution. Further, much of the discourse around automobility and walking is urban-based. In rural areas the car is almost essential for daily life, both for reasons of relative location and poor public transport. Walking is not an option if one is 10 miles from the nearest school.

The benefits to health and well-being are recognised by children themselves, as interesting research in Auckland, New Zealand makes clear (Mitchell et al. 2007). The authors examine (using story-writing and photography) the experiences of 130 children (aged 6-7 and 10-11 years) in their journeys from home to school. The widespread use of the car for travel means that children 'develop an "island geography" comprising locations that they are chauffeured to and from' (Mitchell et al. 2007: 616), restricting the richer experiences of the journey on foot. Children themselves complain about the trip by car being boring, and over 45% express a desire for more active travel. As one put it: 'I would really like to walk the whole way, even if it was raining. Nature is beautiful and I love to look at it' (Mitchell et al. 2007: 620). Others recognise the benefits of social interaction with other children walking to school, and staying healthy: 'I would like to get energy, get healthy and brainy' (p. 620). But Mitchell and her colleagues make the pertinent point that walking to school is not only about children's agency. It is also about the structural constraints that inhibit walking; such constraints include those imposed by parents anxious about safety, the distances separating some homes and schools, but also 'employment-generated routines which mean that adults are driving to work at the same time as children are making their way to school' (Mitchell et al. 2007: 625).

An alternative to having a solitary child walk to school is to promote the 'walking school bus' (WSB), whereby a group of children walk to and from the school under the supervision of a volunteer adult (usually a parent). This idea has taken off in New Zealand cities such as Christchurch and Auckland (Kingham and Ussher 2007; Collins and Kearns 2010). Perceived benefits for participants and parents include creating healthy lifestyles and fitness; in addition 'the children let off steam walking to school (which increases their fitness)…and…they are more settled upon arrival at school' (Collins and Kearns 2010: 5). Further, friendships are developed (and neighbourhood social capital therefore enhanced), car usage is reduced, as are levels of congestion, pollution and accident risk. But evidence from Auckland suggests that take-up of WSBs is uneven, being concentrated more in those schools whose catchments comprise the better-off neighbourhoods.

Some studies (Baig et al. 2009) suggest that individual factors shape active commuting; among children living in deprived parts of the city of Birmingham, UK, white children were much more likely to be active commuters than non-white children, and girls more likely to commute actively than boys. Yet, while walking or cycling to school is beneficial to health, the uptake depends upon perceived safety as well as the distance to be travelled. Further, we cannot expect improved rates of walking or cycling to be the responsibility of individual families; environmental improvements and 'liveable' neighbourhoods are required. Timperio and colleagues (2006), in a study based in Melbourne, Australia, found that neighbourhoods with busy intersections, poor access to lights and street crossings, and routes with relatively steep inclines all inhibited walking or cycling to school. Findings such as these have led to the 'Safe Routes to School' initiative in North America (originating in Marin County, California) that is designed to decrease traffic and pollution and increase the health of children. The programme (www.saferoutestoschools.org/index.shtml) addresses the safety concerns of parents by encouraging greater enforcement of traffic laws and exploring ways to create safer streets.

What evidence is there of the effectiveness of various interventions designed to promote walking, whether by children or adults? TenBrink and his colleagues (2009) have revealed the benefits of having a community-based approach, involving numerous different agencies and organisations in the blue-collar city of Jackson, Michigan. Known as 'Project U-Turn' it sought to address the extraordinarily high levels of obesity in the city (21% of the population estimated to be obese, and 62% overweight). Initiatives included walking school buses and 'smart commuting' (uses of buses, cycling and walking for travel to and from work). Substantial increases in the number of people using active transport were recorded, though interest in the WSB programmes seemed to wane over time. Ogilvie and his colleagues (2007) have reviewed a set of 48 controlled trials of walking interventions, some delivered to the individual, others to households or groups. Interventions that seem to be fairly effective include: brief advice given face to face in the workplace; advice given by telephone or via the internet (see Chapter 10); led walks; provision of pedometers; and mass media campaigns. They suggest that some of these can increase walking among targeted participants (for example, those currently very sedentary) by up to 60 minutes a week, though evidence suggests these increases are difficult to sustain over a longer period. Of the studies that reported a significant increase in walking, several found that self-reported health, wellbeing, and quality of life also improved.

Dumurgier and colleagues (2009) have undertaken interesting research on the association between *speed* of walking and risk of death in older people from the city of Dijon, France. Those persons who had a lower walking speed at the start of the study were at greater risk of death five years after being followed up. Specifically, those in the bottom third of walking speed were 44% more likely than those in the upper third to have died, and there was a threefold increase in risk of death from cardiovascular disease. It was not the case that the slow walkers were already suffering from heart disease. McCarthy (1999), in an overview of transport and health, suggests that regular walking promotes cardiovascular fitness and confers long-term benefits by limiting obesity, strengthening heart muscle and lowering blood pressure. Exercise through walking also reduced the risk of osteoporosis (loss of bone density) that may develop in older adults, particularly women. In a recent longitudinal study of older adults Erickson and colleagues (2010) demonstrated an association between physical activity and the volume of grey matter in brains. Those adults who walked between 6 and 9 miles a week were less likely to have suffered loss of grey matter (compared with their brain volume 9 years earlier) than inactive adults. Further, this activity halved the risk of developing cognitive impairment or the onset of dementia. Clearly, being an active walker well into old age is protective of health.

There is evidence of an association between mobility and perception of neighbourhood safety. Clark and her colleagues (2009) undertook a longitudinal study of a cohort of adults aged over 65 years in 1982 living in New Haven, Connecticut. After eight years follow-up those living below the poverty line perceived neighbourhood safety hazards to a much greater extent than those who were better off, and this had a direct effect on their mobility. As the authors put it, neighbourhoods that are perceived as dangerous 'get into the body' to engender mobility disability. Bennett et al. (2007) report much the same among middle-aged adults living in low-income neighbourhoods in Boston. Perceiving one's neighbourhood as unsafe during the day-time is, for both men and women, associated with significantly less physical activity. Women feeling unsafe at night took over 1000 fewer steps than those who felt safe in their immediate area. This clearly limits, potentially, the effectiveness of physical activity programmes; it may help to provide people with pedometers and exercise programmes, but if the local environment is perceived as unsafe or unattractive the effectiveness of these may well be constrained.

There is a growing body of evidence (in both Canada and Portugal, for example: see Harrington and Elliott 2009; Santana et al. 2009) to suggest that neighbourhood characteristics – such as pedestrian-friendly streets, presence of parks – are at least as important as individual motivation in securing increased amounts of walking and consequent reductions in obesity. Those neighbourhoods with poor layout or facilities, and therefore not conducive to walking, may be considered 'obesogenic'. Neighbourhoods that have high levels of 'walkability' (good levels of street connectivity, high residential density, high land use mix) are associated with higher levels of physical activity (van Dyck et al. 2009). A growing number of studies are using Geographic Information Systems (GIS) techniques to assess walkability (for a detailed example in New York City, see Neckerman et al. 2009). However, GIS-based measures of 'access' to parks and walkable neighbourhoods are rather simple. One might expect that people living in neighbourhoods that are, socio-economically, relatively deprived, would have poorer access to walkable environments. This does not always seem to be the case (Cutts et al. 2009). There is a need to take into account the attractiveness of facilities; the run-down park that is perceived as

Table 2.1   Measures of physical environment in census tracts, New York City

Measure	Non-poor census tracts	Poor census tracts
Density of street trees per sq km	1006	508
Percentage tracts with bicycle racks	24	3
Percentage tracts with sidewalk cafes	16	3

Source: Neckerman et al. (2009).

unsafe is hardly likely to generate much enthusiasm for walking. Equally, 'street connectivity' is measured by the density of intersecting streets (van Dyck et al. 2009) and this seems rather crude; the walk along a single highway that borders a pleasant park may be substantially more appealing than a walk with lots of turns that cuts through a shabby urban environment. Neckerman and her colleagues provide good empirical evidence that this is the case, using both GIS data and field evidence; census tracts in New York City that have high levels of poverty have significantly fewer clean, tree-lined streets, cafes and other features of an attractive street-scape, compared with wealthier neighbourhoods (Table 2.1).

It is increasingly recognised that walking and cycling are good for population health. Guidelines (Shephard 2008) suggest that, in order to reduce the risk of death from cardiovascular disease, people should walk up to 1.9 km in 22 minutes twice a day, for 5 days a week, or cycle at 16 km/hr for 11 minutes twice a day, 5 days a week. For many, especially those living in unattractive environments, these are challenging targets indeed. Workplace initiatives to promote active commuting, such as providing showers and cycle racks, are likely to confer clear benefits. But wider structural and environmental improvements, such as better urban design and provision of dedicated walking/cycling routes, are also required.

It is important to assess the evidence that people are willing to shift mode of transport away from the car to walking and cycling. Ogilvie and his colleagues (2004) have reviewed a number of interventions designed to deliver such modal shift. They found that targeted programmes such as 'Travelsmart' (piloted in Perth, Australia, and in Gloucestershire, UK) contributed to such shift; the programme delivers leaflets, timetables, maps and free bus tickets in a trial period to participants. In Aarhus, Denmark, the 'Bikebusters' programme (giving suburban car commuters a free bicycle and bus pass for one year) led to a 25% shift from car travel. Conversely, car sharing schemes, road charging and publicity campaigns had little impact. In terms of health impact, the 'Walk in to Work Out' experiment in Glasgow showed significant improvements in mental health and vitality after six months (www.pathsforall.org.uk/pathstohealth/workplaceworkout.asp).

An implication from the above is that walking is something to be celebrated, either for its contribution to good health or the fact that the resulting footprints are non-carbon. In some respects it can be constructed as a *choice* to be made by those with health or environmental consciences. Of course, for some people, it is not a choice but a necessity. I shall leave to Chapter 6 a discussion of the walking that is forced on the dispossessed. But I wish to say something here about the experience of groups in the global north for whom walking is compulsory because they do not own, or have access to, a car.

In Britain there is a wide disparity, according to income, between those households with and without a car; less than one-third of low income households with children have access to a car. Buses might be used, but for those on low incomes they are an additional cost to be borne. The travel constraints imposed on non car-owning households have been explored carefully by Bostock (2001), who has looked at the experiences of 30 mothers with small children, living on low incomes in central England. She suggests that there are three ways in which such women are disadvantaged.

The first is that they struggle to manage the demands of pre-school children who are walking with them. The women in Bostock's sample described the difficulties of getting small children ready and the hazards of walking with them along busy roads. Others refer directly to the hazard of the road: 'Crossing the road is such a worry. The roads round here are just so busy. It makes life so stressful' (Bostock, 2001: 15). A second source of disadvantage, and health-related problem, is that the women themselves are fatigued by the journey on foot. As one puts it: 'there's me with a bloody pushchair full, sky-high with shopping and trying to push up the road. It would be nice just to dump it in the car and come home, you know' (Bostock 2001: 14). For another: 'I suppose that it could be good exercise for me but quite honestly it's just such a burden' (Bostock 2001: 15). The third source of disadvantage is the spatial constraint that restricts their range and ties them to areas that are lacking in resources and infrastructure. The spatial concentration of food stores, and primary and secondary health care, means that those without cars have to use a combination of walking and public transport to access such resources. Those in employment have also to negotiate time off work, which is compounded by extra journey times. These spatial constraints deny these women access to the social and network capital so prized in the mobilities literature. Bostock's study reveals very neatly the contrast with those who have the choice to walk or who are keen to encourage 'the public' to do so. For other people, life is not so simple. This is also true in the global south, where the gender disparities often far wider. In an ethnographic study of two commuters in Santiago, Chile, Jirón (2009: 128) paints a vivid picture of the commuting undertaken by a female domestic cleaner, whose travel experience on two buses is one of being in considerable discomfort and some danger. For her, mobility is hardly liberating; rather, she is confined in a mobile place. Network capital is in short supply.

There are other dangers in walking, not least those suffered by the vulnerable late at night. The media frequently carry stories of women targeted by unscrupulous taxi (cab) drivers or accosted and perhaps assaulted as they make their way home, alone, after a night out. Urry (2007: 74) refers to the 'interactional vandalism' that may be directed at women, older people and people of colour. 'Roughly speaking the more diverse the others walking about, the safer the environment' (Urry 2007: 74).

On your bike

Ownership of mass-produced bicycles became more common in the early 20th century and led to the growth of cycling as a recreational activity. 'This new form of recreation could be enjoyed by the lone rider but the camaraderie of the local cycling club was also a key feature of the fashion, especially among young men' (Aitchison et al. 2000: 43). It freed people from the constraints of the public transport timetable and, away from the city, provided a cheap way of leaving behind the air-polluted city and inhaling cleaner air. How popular is it in contemporary society, and what are the health benefits?

Pucher and Buehler (2008) have offered a very good answer to the first question, revealing the success of public policy in Denmark, the Netherlands, and Germany in encouraging cycling, compared with the US and UK. Their data (Table 2.2) reveal the propensity for making trips (and short-distance trips in particular) by bicycle in the Netherlands and Denmark. While only one-quarter of cyclists in the UK and US are women, the proportions are about half in the other three countries.

Broad national variations mask variability within countries. For example, in the Netherlands the percentage of trips made by bicycle is 37% in Groningen but only 16% in Rotterdam. In Copenhagen and Aalborg (Denmark) the percentages are 29% and 17% respectively, and in Munster and Stuttgart, Germany, the figures are 27% and 6%. In none of the Canadian and American cities the authors list do the figures exceed 5%. Pucher and Buehler (2008) ascribe these differences to the more bicycle-sensitive transport, land-use, housing, environmental, taxation and parking policies adopted in the Netherlands, Denmark and Germany. Dutch, Danish and German cities are people-friendly rather than car-friendly, hence more liveable and sustainable than those in Britain and the US (Pucher and Buehler 2008: 496).

Over time, cycling as a proportion of trips made has declined, though this decline was arrested during the mid-1970s as transport and land-use policy shifted in the three continental European cities studied by Pucher and Buehler. Horton and his colleagues (2007: 3) suggest that 37% of all journeys were by bicycle in 1949, compared with 1% in 2001; even in Beijing, China, the percentage has dropped from 60% to 40% since the turn of the century. However, more recent evidence suggests that cycle use is on the rise, partly to address environmental sustainability concerns, but also health ones. Cycling benefits individuals, but also organisations that do not have to tie up resources with expensive car parking spaces (Horton et al. 2007: 6-7). The benefits may be quite intangible; perhaps car users and passengers can enjoy their own rides but – away from the city centre – the cyclist can indulge senses other than the solely visual. Sometimes the pleasures can be enjoyed in the

Table 2.2   Cycling in Europe and the USA: volume and risk

	Netherlands	Denmark	Germany	UK	USA
Percentage of total trips by bicycle	27	18	10	1	1
Kilometres cycled per inhabitant per day	2.5	1.6	0.9	0.2	0.1
Percentage of trips, less than 2.5 km, made by bicycle	37	27	14	2	2
Percentage of bicycle trips made by women	55	45	49	29	25
Cyclists killed per 100 million km cycled	1.1	1.5	1.7	3.6	5.8
Cyclists injured per 10 million km cycled	1.4	1.7	4.7	6.0	37.5

Source: All data taken from graphs in Pucher and Buehler (2008).

company of other cyclists; often they are solitary ones. McBeth (2009: 173) relates a memoir of one cyclist: 'Riding solo always had a pleasant melancholy aspect for me. Some days I was happy to be alone with my thoughts, and for the sights and sounds and scents of those lanes to belong to me...by the time I had turned for home, though, I always found my mood lightened'.

Of course, if cycling is to be promoted properly, policies need to attend to devising a comprehensive network of cycle routes; routes that are reasonably direct, attractive and safe. Such a network was established in the UK in 1995. The National Cycle Network is a comprehensive network of cycle routes, comprising some 12000 miles, one third of which is on traffic-free paths, with the remainder on quiet lanes or traffic-calmed roads. See www.sustrans.org.uk/what-we-do/national-cycle-network. The network is primarily used for recreational purposes, with 25% of users citing health or fitness as reasons for using it (Parkin et al. 2007: 73). Even without such a national network the use of former railway lines and canal tow-paths offers good opportunities for recreational cycling. However, the availability of such cycle-friendly initiatives can make roads seem even more out of place for the cyclist.

Cyclists are at times highly visible, and at other times highly invisible, road users. They are visible when they appear to impinge on the 'rights' of other road users and (as Horton 2007 notes) for some women the bicycle does nothing to shield them from the masculine gaze. They are invisible to the thoughtless car driver. Thus, cyclists are exposed to various sources of risk in the environment, whether from car drivers, other cyclists, or pedestrians.

There are risks to the cyclist from the drivers on the roads. Naci and colleagues (2009) estimate that there are about 107,000 deaths of cyclists each year, with the vast majority of these occurring in low- and middle-income countries. Fifteen per cent of casualties in China are cyclists. Such risks are clearly a deterrent to would-be cyclists and, as Horton (2007: 135) observes, may explain why some prefer the safety of the pedalling machine in the gym or home. Fear, as Horton (2007) puts it, has driven cyclists off the road, and as fewer cyclists remain the more 'out of place' they appear to be and the more exposed they are to risk. Pucher and Buehler (2008) assert there is safety in numbers, with lower fatality and injury rates in countries with higher bicycling shares of travel. Well-meaning policies, particularly those directed towards children, do little to help. Rather than promoting positive images of cycling the campaigns (particularly on television) convey an impression of danger and accident.

Interviews with 100 cyclists in Cambridge conducted by Skinner and Rosen (2007) suggest that other cyclists are sometimes to blame. Some of these 'cycle at night without lights, they move around on the road unpredictably and without indicating, they ride the wrong way up one-way streets – and because of this they give all cyclists a bad name' (Skinner and Rosen 2007: 92). Thus, not infrequently, cyclists have at times to endure stereotyping by those on four wheels; 'in Britain, cyclists tend to be caricatured as lycra-clad louts, self-righteous eco-warriors, freeloaders (because they travel on roads without paying road tax) and serial ignorers of red lights' (Moran 2009: 117).

What impact does legislation have on the wearing of bicycle helmets? Legislation exists in Australia, New Zealand, Canada and the US – but not in the UK. Studies have examined both the wearing of helmets and also the impact on injury rates. In an interesting study Pardi and colleagues (2007) showed a 27% reduction in injury rates to cyclists aged under 16 years, one year after the introduction of legislation in the US, a reduction that remained at 24% five years later. A meta-analysis of literature on whether wearing helmets reduces the risk of death or serious head injury for motorcycle crash victims suggests strong evidence in favour. Liu et al. (2008) indicate that the risk of death is reduced by 42%, and the risk of serious head injury by 69%. This is supported by a Cochrane review (Macpherson and Spinks 2008) which found evidence to suggest that legislation both increases helmet use and reduces bicycle-related head injuries. But there is evidence that helmet use depends upon context. Kakefuda and colleagues (2009) found that while 37% of student cyclists in a Colorado university wore helmets while riding recreationally, only 9% did when commuting to campus, in part because of the shorter distances involved and the perception of reduced risk.

In the continental European countries studied by Pucher and Buehler (2008) – the Netherlands, Denmark and Germany – helmet wearing is not compulsory. Only 1% of adults, and less than 5% of children in the Netherlands, wear helmets. Rates of helmet use are higher in Denmark and Germany (66% and 33% of children aged 6-10 years wear helmets). As we saw earlier (Table 2.2) fatality rates among cyclists in all three countries are low, though the injury rates among German cyclists are much higher than in the other two countries. All these figures are related, according to Pucher and Buehler, to the physical separation of cyclists from motorised traffic, via cycle paths and lanes, and to traffic calming schemes that restrict the speed of cars and other vehicles.

Arguments for and against the wearing of helmets (and the benefits or otherwise of legislation to enforce their wearing) tend to be quite polarised. Robinson (2006) suggests that forcing unwilling cyclists to don helmets deters them from cycling and therefore negates the physical health benefits they would otherwise enjoy. She also invokes the risk compensation hypothesis to suggest that motorists take less care if they see a helmeted cyclist and that cyclists themselves are more prone to risky behaviours on the road if they wear a helmet. Her argument is that legislation in Australia has delivered no significant reduction in head injuries. But Hagel and his colleagues (2006) have taken issue with this; before the helmet law was introduced in New South Wales bicycle-related head injuries dropped by about 1% in the previous two years, but by 4.3% immediately after.

Canadian research has examined socio-economic gradients in bicycle helmet use among children aged 5-14 years (Parkin et al. 2003; Macpherson et al. 2006). Legislation was introduced in 1995 requiring helmets to be worn. In the study area of East York, Toronto, observations of children riding showed that helmet use rose overall from 44% before legislation to 68% after but that children in high-income neighbourhoods were more likely to wear them. Helmet use rose in low and medium-income areas from 33% and 50% to 61% and 79% respectively. However, six years after the introduction of legislation observational data suggested that helmet use in low and medium-income areas had returned to pre-legislation levels, while use in high-income areas had been maintained at around 75% (Macpherson et al. 2006).

All I need is the air that I breathe

Those walking in urban environments, along or near busy roads, are exposed to vehicle exhaust emissions; nitrogen dioxide and particulates are the pollutants most clearly linked to road transport. This kind of exposure can be assessed crudely by examining whether or not people live on routes carrying various levels of traffic. Or, it can be determined by modelling the likely burden of pollution, drawing on a set of fixed monitoring sites in urban areas and then interpolating from these to estimate the pollution load at any other location; this is of course subject to sampling and statistical error. Neither of these approaches suffices if one wishes to assess personal exposure. Consequently, some authors have explored the use of personal monitoring devices. Greaves et al. (2008) used such monitors to assess exposure to fine particulates in streets of varying traffic densities in Sydney, Australia. Fine particulates are of interest because they can penetrate deep into the lungs, causing potentially serious respiratory disease. Greaves and colleagues' work is important because it can assess exposures that are not merely background ('ambient') but are spatially and temporally very specific. Their work reveals second-by-second exposures and links these to specific 'hot-spots' such as busy intersections or the behaviour of particular vehicles. All this detail is masked by averages that are usually estimated in research of this kind.

The use of such personal monitoring devices is not unproblematic, in part because of the cost involved. Rather than fit individuals with such monitors, other researchers prefer to collect detailed data on where people spend their time and under what conditions of exposure to particular kinds of pollutant. This so-called 'activity-based modelling' clearly draws on the ideas of time-space geography considered in Chapter 1.

In an interesting study, Davies and Whyatt (2009) seek to determine optimal pedestrian (or cycle) paths for school-age children that minimise exposure to environmental pollution. Such paths could then be compared with those that are conventionally taken by the children. Using a standard air dispersion model to depict a pollution surface in a built-up area they use Geographic Information Systems (GIS) methods to determine that route from a school to a child's home address which minimises total distance travelled and exposure to pollution. GPS data are used to provide information on the routes actually taken by children. The results suggest alternative routes that might be taken to avoid pollution exposure whilst also allowing for journey length. If we are to encourage walking to school this kind of approach could pay real dividends. More ambitiously, as the authors note, 'location-specific advice on low exposure routes could be streamed direct to a mobile phone providing individuals with the opportunity to make informed decisions in real-time' (Davies and Whyatt 2009: 243).

This work is all the more significant in view of research undertaken by Briggs and his colleagues (2008), and others, which seeks to assess the differing exposures from alternate travel modes. In a study conducted in London the authors compared exposures to particulate pollution (thought to be the main health risk) from those journeying on foot and those travelling by car, along the same 46 routes and at the same time. The average exposures along all routes are between 2 and almost 5 times higher for walking compared with in-car travel; however, examining the cumulative exposures (which take into account the different journey times) the differences are almost 16-fold for the coarse particulates (Table 2.3). As the authors observe, breathing rates while on foot are likely to be greater than in the vehicle, simply because of increased physiological activity. The inferences are clear, and sobering for public health policy. The benefits of encouraging walking will only be realised if policies are implemented that separate, more than at present, road vehicles and pedestrians (also cyclists); dedicated and convenient walking and cycling routes are required (Briggs et al. 2008: 21).

Precisely the same conclusion is reached by Int Panis and his colleagues (2010) in a study of exposure to particulates among cyclists and car passengers in Belgium. The importance of this study lies in the very detailed measurement of particulate concentrations to which people are exposed in the car and on the bicycle but, in addition, simultaneous respiratory measurements of both sets. This allowed them to assess the health effects of short bursts of high exposure to pollutants. Looking at car users and cyclists in three Belgian locations (Brussels, Louvain

Table 2.3   **Mean cumulative exposures to particulates on foot and in-car, London**

Particulate size	In-car	Walking	Ratio
Coarse	22.83	356.6	15.62
Fine	11.61	86.16	7.42
Very fine	6.82	44.26	6.49

Source: Briggs et al. (2008): 19.

and Mol) their results (Table 2.4) suggest that the average inhaled quantities of fine particulates (PM2.5) are considerably higher for the cyclists, because of the greater inhaled volume of air. Cyclists appear to be exposed at least six times more than car passengers. Of course, as the authors note, the physical activity undertaken by cyclists is protective of chronic conditions such as heart disease.

Table 2.4   **Average inhaled quantity of fine particulates (PM2.5) in three Belgian locations**

Location	Mode	PM2.5 inhaled (μg/km)
Brussels	Bike	3.4
	Car	0.6
	Bike/car ratio	5.9
Louvain	Bike	3.8
	Car	0.5
	Bike/car ratio	8.0
Mol	Bike	5.2
	Car	0.7
	Bike/car ratio	7.4

Source: Int Panis et al. (2010): 2267.

Rather than restricting cycling, the policy suggestion is (as in Briggs' study) to separate the modes of transport and reduce the exposure of cyclists to pollutants.

Having looked at the possible means of assessing exposure, what do we know about the possible health consequences of inhaling contaminants? There is a very large literature in environmental epidemiology on this subject, with effects ranging from respiratory problems, asthma, some cancers, and heart disease. Let me focus on impacts on child health.

Gauderman and his colleagues (2007) studied the impact on the health of children in California (aged 10-18 years) of proximity to highways (freeways). The authors measured the lung function of over 3500 children, each year, and related this to how far the children lived from the nearest major road. After adjusting for socio-economic circumstances (one might expect poorer children to have worse lung function) the authors found that children living within 500m of a freeway had significantly worse lung function than those living progressively further away. This is an indirect measure of 'exposure', but nonetheless the impact on child health is quite clear. A more direct measure of exposure is used by McConnell and his colleagues (2010) in a further study of child respiratory health in Southern California. Concentrations of pollutants from vehicle emissions were estimated at both children's homes and their schools, using air dispersion models. Using a cohort of over 5300 children aged about 6 years, the authors followed up their health to see which developed asthma. The risk of developing asthma was significantly associated with traffic-related pollution near both the home and the school (where children spend much of their time). Given that about 10% of schools in California are located within 150 m of major roads – those with at least 25,000 vehicles each day – the potential pollution burden and health risks cannot be over-estimated. The cost of such disease is both social and economic; the demand on health services goes up, as do school absences. The impact on the families and the children themselves will be considerable.

Other studies have examined the impact of traffic-related air pollution on children's cognitive and neurological functioning. Wang and colleagues (2009) examined children in two schools in Quanzhou, China, one of which was located in a polluted area with high traffic density, the other in an area with few roads and good air quality. Using a number of standard tests of neuro-behavioural performance (including reaction times) on samples of over 400 children in each school, results showed that children in the polluted area had significantly poorer performance on most tests than those in the less polluted area, after appropriate adjustment for confounding factors.

Concluding remarks

While walking and cycling can be hazardous occupations – though often only hazardous because of the behaviour of others – there is plenty of evidence to suggest they are health-promoting. Considerable research has been undertaken on the medical benefits of both leisure-time physical activity, including walking and cycling, and the benefits of active commuting. In particular, the protective effects of such activity on cardiovascular disease, particularly when undertaken in relatively short bursts, is well-established (Hamer and Chida 2008). Overall, it appears that active commuting reduces the risk of cardiovascular disease by 11%, after adjusting for possible confounding effects (such as the likelihood that active commuters may be more 'active' in general). The reduced risk of cardiovascular disease appears slightly more marked for women than for men (Hu et al. 2007). In contrast, men appear to have better *mental health* outcomes than women who engage in active commuting. A study of 670 office workers in Japan (Ohta et al. 2007) found that mental health in the male cohort improved steadily according to time spent in commuting to work on foot or bicycle, an effect that was not detected for female workers. But these health improvements have to be set against the negative impacts of walking and cycling in risky and potentially polluted environments.

Jacobsen and colleagues (2009) document the evidence that people avoid dangerous and unpleasant traffic. The consequences of such avoidance are obvious; people will walk and cycle less and their health and fitness will suffer, contributing to the obesity 'epidemic' that has been witnessed in recent years. The car has appropriated spaces that were, 50 years ago, adopted by children for play. Health policy in Europe and the US suggests that adults should engage in at least 30 minutes of physical activity each day (children at least 60 minutes); clearly, walking/cycling to work/school could make a major contribution to reaching these targets. Evidence suggests that only about a third of the population reach such targets. One explanation is the fear induced by injury prevention campaigns, which stress that the responsibility for accidents lies with the incautious pedestrian or cyclist rather than the car driver. The (potential) victims are blamed. Even the terminology (of a road traffic *accident*) suggests that blame lies less with the person in charge of the motorised vehicle and more with the careless other. I return to this issue in the next chapter.

Walking and cycling invariably slow things down and give us (back) time. Paul Tranter (2010) has drawn attention to the work of Carl Honoré, whose book 'In Praise of Slow' espouses the adoption of a slower pace of life. Tranter also reminds us of the 'Slow Cities' initiative (part of the Slow Movement: www.slowmovement. com) that seeks to encourage use of local products and food, reducing the need for transport but also encouraging a slower pace of life. As Tranter suggests, lack of time, and the pursuit of speed, is becoming a major public health issue, as people consume fast(er) food and find less time to engage in healthy pursuits. I turn now to the costs and benefits, to individual and public health, of using faster travel.

Chapter 3
Four Wheels Good?

Introduction

The title of this chapter borrows from George Orwell's classic novel *Animal Farm* in which, as the animals drive out the farmer, their motto is 'Four legs good, two legs bad'; the animals are good and their two-legged human oppressors are bad. Whether four wheels are better – or much worse – than two wheels is the focus of the chapter.

There has been very large growth in the volume of vehicles on roads, and distance travelled, across the world. For example, in 1970 cars in the US travelled some 920 billion miles, but by 2004 this had risen to 1705 billion miles (Gatrell and Elliott 2009: 190). In Britain in 1930 there were 2.3 million motor vehicles on the road, rising to 15 million by 1970 and more than doubling over the last 40 years to 34.2 million (Office for National Statistics 2010). Also in Britain there has been a steady rise, since the 1970s, in the proportion of households with two cars; 27% of households now have two cars, while 7% of households have three or more. Of course, this is geographically differentiated; while almost half (47%) of households in rural areas had two or more cars, the proportion in London was 17%. Travel by local bus has fallen dramatically since 1955, from 15.6 million journeys to 5.2 million in 2008.

How does travel on four wheels relate to human health and well-being? I begin by exploring the ways in which the car contributes to a sense of well-being. For the driver and any passengers the trip can engender benefits to mental health. But these benefits are set against many risks, risks encountered by both the car's occupants and other road users, pedestrians, or those living near roads. Some of these were touched on in the previous chapter. The car is not the only motorised vehicle of interest, however. While they (usually) have more than four wheels I shall also consider the health impacts, on both occupants and others, of buses and trucks (lorries).

The pleasures of driving

As Urry (2007: 119) notes, cars can be seen as liberating and offering 'privatized flexibility'. Canzler (2008: 105) suggests that for 'all their unintended side effects, such as traffic jams, scarce parking and accidents, they broaden the individual's optional spaces of mobility'. In contrast to public transport, they offer independence and control. Many advertisements make much of the pleasurable aspects of the open road (they rarely show their cars stationary in traffic jams; rather, in quite exotic environments). While they involve expense in purchase and maintenance, taxation and insurance, assuming one has a valid licence they do not require permission to drive, or the purchase of a ticket.

Urry (2007: 120) refers to the car journey as 'being encapsulated in a domestic, cocooned, moving capsule'. Moran (2009: 94) suggests that the modern car is 'a projection of status and bravado, a *mobile personal space* within which motorists could feel both embattled and emboldened' (my italics). It confers status, autonomy and control. We might suggest the car-owner possesses symbolic capital (even network capital) as cars allow the user more 'spatial reach' and flexibility than does perhaps public transport (Ellaway et al. 2003).

Not being able to drive, or having access to a car can be a considerable disadvantage. Consuming the car becomes almost essential to the smooth operation of contemporary social life; it is 'naturalized and embedded in everyday life – psychically, socially, culturally and materially' (Freund and Martin, 2001: 203). Transport (and social and cultural life) remains fundamentally car-centred, to the neglect of other forms of movement. But those who emphasise the sociality of walking may forget that the car journey can also be a social activity, either for the parent/s and child/ren who share a journey or for commuters who car-share. Friendships can be developed in the car as well as on foot. Of course, any parent will recognise that travelling with young children (who may be restless and demand frequent stops on long journeys) can be stressful rather than pleasurable!

In the interwar period (the 1920s and 1930s) using the car for leisure trips became firmly established for those in the western world who could afford access. Peters (2006: Chapter 4) traces the growth of 'auto camps' in the US and the emergence of the motel as a more comfortable stop. Even today the car is, in the developed world, a means of helping some of us escape the city for the countryside, perhaps for day trips or (for the well-off) for a weekend in the country. In making such trips we do not necessarily take the most direct route; we may take a more circuitous route if we feel the journey will be more interesting and pleasurable. As we see later, for others the car is less of an enabler to access the environment and more a destroyer of such environments.

Sheller (2004) explores the experience of 'dwelling with cars' and the set of 'emotional investments' in the car. She reminds us that the very language of emotion is inflected with mobility metaphors; we are 'moved' or 'transported' by events; we might even go on a 'trip'. Many of the automotive emotions are positive. She quotes a colleague: 'Whilst I am driving, I am nearly always happy. Driving towards virtually anywhere makes me excited, expectant: full of hope' (Sheller 2004: 224). For some, the very act of owning (and perhaps naming) a car makes them feel good, depending on the state of the vehicle and how often it lets them down. But Sheller reminds us there is potential frustration and pain in the trip too. The movement of the car is pleasurable for some but not for the child with motion sickness.

The way in which ownership of a car can confer psycho-social benefits in a way that contrasts with public transport has been explored by researchers in Glasgow (Hiscock et al. 2002; Ellaway et al. 2003). The authors suggest that people remain attached to cars because of the prestige, protection and autonomy (a set of attributes that is labelled 'ontological security') that they provide. Because of this they suggest that cars can be health-promoting. Other work they have done in the west of Scotland suggests that mental and physical health was better among car owners than others, independent of income, sex and age. The ontological security afforded by cars, and thus attachment to them, means that there is an uphill battle to shift people away from car travel. Public transport is seen by respondents as lacking in protection from unpleasant conditions or threatening situations (such as waiting in a cold, wet or windy place for a bus or train, or waiting at night in a poorly lit place). Public transport is also seen by many as unreliable or not taking people directly to their destination. As one of Hiscock's respondents puts it: 'I enjoy the privacy of the car. It's like an extension of your own personal space, whereas in public transport...you tend to get your space invaded because everybody's packed in, close knit, which sometimes can be – if you're not in a good mood, it can be quite off-putting really, and *it can maybe raise your stress levels*'. (Hiscock et al. 2002: 125, my italics). The car provides 'a sanctuary, a zone of protection, however slender, between oneself and the surrounding transport environment' (Lyons and Urry 2005: 265).

Context is all important; whether a trip to the busy recycling plant engenders the same *affect* (emotion) as a trip to the garden centre for plants is a moot point. Just as the mental health benefits of a walk depend on time of day and the interest of the route, so too (for me) a motorway journey on the M6, north of Lancaster towards Carlisle, passing the Howgill Fells and the fringes of the Lake District, is very much more pleasurable than driving along the M6 further south, as it nears Birmingham in the post-industrial landscape of the West Midlands. Volume of traffic matters a great deal; a car trip along sparse rural roads has more appeal than rush-hour journeys.

Moran (2009: 113) refers to the communities that can develop on the road, especially among lorry (truck drivers). 'Even on the vast, lonely sea of the motorway, we still find solace in the idea of community'. We might expect, in principle, to see such 'communities' develop among groups of individuals commuting to work by train from the same station, but this does not seem to be the case. Moreover, some will prefer their own company, in their car; as a former UK transport Minister remarked (a touch sardonically), as such 'you don't have to put up with the dreadful human beings sitting alongside you' (cited in Moran 2009: 229).

One visibly (and often intermittently) mobile group on the road are gypsies and travellers, a marginalised population that is known to have worse health outcomes, and poorer access to health services, than the more settled white population in the UK (Peters et al. 2009). Using in-depth interviews van Cleemput and his colleagues (2007) have explored some of the health-related beliefs and experiences of these frequently-mobile groups. The 27 interviewees all described their health in relation to their ability to travel. Even though some lived in, or had experience of, more settled domestic environments all had experienced the traditional travelling lifestyle which is a way of life for many. Most related the health-related benefits from the 'travelling way'; these include freedom and choice, fresh air, proximity to extended family members. But others spoke of the hostility from members of the wider public, a diminishing choice of resting places, and poor access to services. Some felt imprisoned on rented sites and many had low expectations of health. For example, one woman suggested that 'my health is perfect, lovely...I only have a bad back all the time – that's since I was 15' (quoted in van Cleemput et al. 2007: 208).

Road traffic 'accidents'

Set against the car's benefits are risks, both to individual car users and those with whom they interact. So let me discuss at some length one of the most visible dis-benefits conferred on society and individuals by the automobile – the car crash. Car crashes are commonly referred to as 'road traffic accidents' (RTAs), though as some authors (Urry 2007: 118) are keen to point out they are not so much 'accidental' as an inevitable consequence of our living in an 'auto-risk' society. Consequently, I shall refer to them below as road traffic *crashes* (RTCs), though this too is an imperfect label, implying simply that one machine crashes into another.

The broad context is that, worldwide, some 50 million people are injured annually, and about 1.27 million die each year as a result of RTCs, making this the 10th leading cause of death. The distribution of this appalling burden is highly uneven globally (Naci et al. 2009). For example, the mortality rate in Iran is 44 per 100,000, compared with 15 and 5 per 100,000 in the USA and UK respectively (Labinjo et al. 2009; Bhalla et al. 2009: 151). Among males aged 15-44 years, 44% of all deaths in Iran are due to RTCs, an extraordinarily high proportion. In Africa the annual death rate from road traffic crashes is estimated at 28.3 per 100,000 (Labinjo et al. 2009). Pirie (2009a: 24) expresses this in an appropriate way, revealing that about 10% of the global 1.27 million deaths occur in sub-Saharan Africa, when that region only has 4% of the world's registered road vehicles.

In 1998, more than 85% of all deaths due to RTCs were in low-income and middle-income countries. This is due primarily to the growth in volume of motor vehicle traffic in such countries, particularly in those undergoing rapid urbanisation. Naci et al. (2009) estimate that 45% of fatalities in low-income countries (those where per capita income is under $905) are pedestrians; for middle-income countries ($906-$11,115) the estimate is 29% and for high-income countries the figure is 18%. This translates into a quarter of a million pedestrian deaths each year in low-income countries and over 160,000 in middle-income countries (Figure 3.1). In Ethiopia 84%, and in Ivory Coast 75% of fatalities are

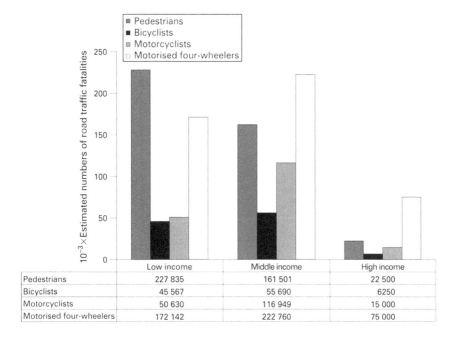

	Low income	Middle income	High income
Pedestrians	227 835	161 501	22 500
Bicyclists	45 567	55 690	6250
Motorcyclists	50 630	116 949	15 000
Motorised four-wheelers	172 142	222 760	75 000

Figure 3.1   Estimated annual number of road traffic deaths, by type of road user and country income

Source: Reprinted with permission from Naci et al. (2009): 58.

pedestrians. Such mortality is, of course, socially patterned, since the poorest, non car owners are those most exposed to such danger.

While pedestrians and cyclists together account for 'only' 23% of RTC deaths in high-income countries, some 72% of deaths are to those in cars or on motorcycles (Naci et al. 2009). This contrasts with 44% in low-income countries and 61% in middle-income countries. Motorcyclists bear the heaviest burden of mortality and injury in south-east Asia and Nigeria, where 54% of RTC injuries are to motorcyclists (Labinjo et al. 2009). Across the globe, some 183,000 motorcyclists are estimated to die each year. Death rates in England and Wales in 2003 were 0.27 per 10 million passenger miles for pedestrians and 0.55 for cyclists. The rate for car occupants was 0.01. Clearly, cyclists and walkers are many times more at risk from accidents than car passengers. As Sonkin and her colleagues observe (2006: 402) 'fear of pedestrian injury can create a vicious circle if an increasingly dangerous pedestrian environment encourages greater car use, leading to higher motorized traffic volumes and greater risks to pedestrians'.

How have rates of RTCs changed over time? Jacobsen and his colleagues (2009) note that US public health officials were keen to trumpet the reduction in fatalities over the 40-year period 1965-2005; but this decline may simply mirror the lower levels of exposure to risk, through much reduced levels of walking and

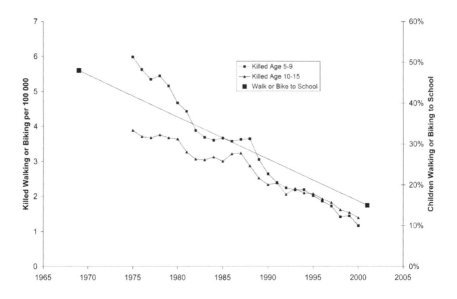

Figure 3.2   School-age children in the USA: safer streets or less walking and cycling?

Source: Reprinted with permission from Jacobsen et al. (2009): 371.

cycling (Figure 3.2). Among the G7 industrial market economies the US has had the highest death rates on the road over the past 25 years, with the UK among the lowest. France has shown a steep decline (Table 3.1).

Table 3.1   Road deaths: G7 comparison (rates per 100,000 population)

	1988	2003	2008
USA	15.4	14.8	12.3
Italy	11.9	11.7	7.9
Canada	9.7	8.7	7.3
France	15.2	10.2	6.9
Germany	9.5	8.0	5.5
Japan	5.5	7.0	4.7
United Kingdom	6.1	6.1	4.3

Source: Office for National Statistics (2010): 14.

Looked at over a longer period we can see the changing proportions of deaths among different road users in Britain (Table 3.2). In 1930 half of all deaths were pedestrians and just over 10% were car drivers and passengers. By 2008 the proportions were 23% and 54% respectively, reflecting in the main the increase in vehicle ownership and the shifting patterns of modal class.

Table 3.2   Road users killed in Britain (percentages)

	1930	1970	2008
Pedestrians	51	39	23
Motorcyclists	25	10	19
Cyclists	12	5	5
Car users	12	46	54

Source: Office for National Statistics (2010): 14.

To what extent are RTCs socially patterned? In the global north there are clear inequalities by social group in the incidence of RTCs and the associated injuries that derive from these. In a study of deaths from injury (including as a result of road incidents) in England and Wales Edwards and his colleagues (2006) observed huge variations in death rates between children whose fathers were employed in professional and managerial occupations, compared with those whose fathers had been unemployed long-term (Table 3.3). Although the numbers of deaths are quite small those children living in households where the father is unemployed are over 20 times more likely to be killed – whether as pedestrians or cyclists – as those where the father works in a high status occupation. Ethnicity ('race') provides another dimension of inequality. In London the average annual pedestrian injury rate, between 1996 and 2006, for children defined as 'black' was 176 per 100,000; but the rates for children of white or 'Asian' background were much lower: 118 and 91 per 100,000 respectively (Steinbach et al. 2010).

Table 3.3   Child death rates from RTC injury in England and Wales, 2001-3

Socio-economic status (father)	Pedestrians		Car occupants		Cyclists	
	No.	Rate	No.	Rate	No.	Rate
Professional/managerial	10	0.2	19	0.4	2	0.05
Long-term unemployed	71	4.7	36	2.4	19	1.3
Ratio of rates		20.6		5.5		27.5

Source: Edwards et al. (2006).
Note: Rates are per 100,000 children aged 0–15, per year.

In the inequalities literature car ownership is invariably regarded as a marker of wealth (and lack thereof has formed one of the components of 'deprivation indices' that have remained in vogue for more than 25 years). Woodcock and Aldred (2008) seek to go beyond this narrow conceptualisation and to locate car ownership within 'the growing global system of corporate commodity production'. They acknowledge that, 'downstream', car ownership causes air

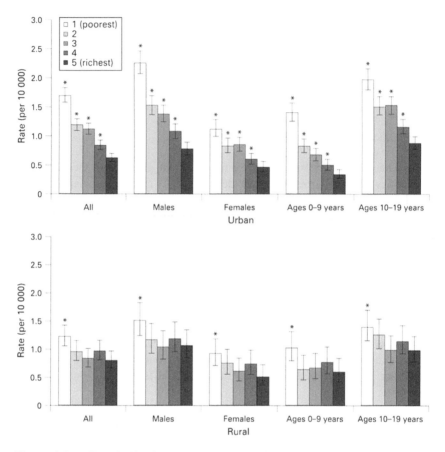

**Figure 3.3   Hospitalisation rates for pedestrians or cyclists injured in a
road traffic accident, by neighbourhood income and urban/
rural residence, Canadian children aged 0-19 years, 2001-05**

Source: Reprinted with permission from Oliver and Kohen (2009): 167.

pollution, noise, injury and mortality, obesity, and reduced social capital, all of
which are socially patterned with burdens falling most acutely on disadvantaged
individuals and groups. But their structuralist interpretation asserts that cars, and
the resource-intensive (oil, rubber, steel) systems into which they are locked,
are 'central to the accumulation strategies of the corporate-dominated global
economy'. The major oil and car corporations have huge budgets for promoting
the car economy, while those trying to improve road safety favour education
over regulation. Putting the onus on the pedestrian (and driver) to be observant
is cheaper, though less effective, than, requiring cars to travel more slowly.
Woodcock and Aldred are critical of this targeting of the powerless, demanding
a focus instead on more powerful corporations and individuals.

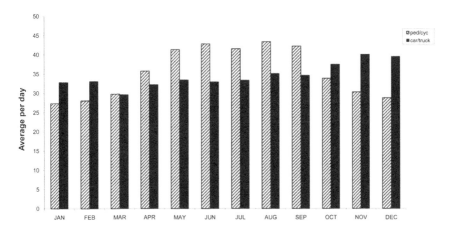

Figure 3.4   Monthly variations in hospital admission, by type of road user, England, 1999-2004

Source: Reprinted with permission from Gill and Goldacre (2009): 376.

For Woodcock and Aldred the violence of the car comes not merely from the prospect of serious injury or fatality but also from what Bourdieu might have called the 'ordinary suffering' due to noisy and polluting engines revving and drivers' impatience with slow pedestrians. Car crime gets constructed as crime *against* the car (theft, break-in) rather than *by* the car (labelled as driving offences or violations). For these authors this violence gets embodied through obesity and cardiovascular disease that results from being too sedentary. The hijacking of urban space for and by the motor car has further negative consequences for social engagement in neighbourhoods.

Oliver and Kohen (2009) looked at the patterns among accidents to children (under 19 years of age) in urban and rural parts of Canada. In rural areas there was some evidence of a gradient in hospitalisation rates for pedestrians and cyclists, but this gradient was sharply pronounced in urban areas, whether for boys or girls, young or older children (Figure 3.3). This may be because of the greater frequency of hazards, such as high traffic levels, poor pavements (sidewalks), and fewer crossing places in low income neighbourhoods. As the authors put it 'the burden of motor vehicle traffic injury hospitalisation is not shared equally among all children' (Oliver and Kohen 2009: 167). The same point has been made by other authors, in other settings. For example, Kim et al. (2007), although studying childhood deaths from injuries as a whole (in which transport-related injuries are only one component), find that the characteristics of districts in Korea influence mortality rates over and above the role played by individual factors. There is a clear gradient in risk according to the material deprivation in such districts; children in the most deprived districts are 50% more likely to die from transport-related injuries than those in the most affluent Korean districts.

What evidence is there on seasonal variation in injury and mortality due to road traffic? Gill and Goldacre (2009) have analysed data for England between 1999 and 2004, observing, as one might expect, a significant summer peak for motorcyclists and cyclists, relatively high levels of injuries to pedestrians and cyclists in summer months (Figure 3.4). Once allowance is made for numbers of trips, cycling is much more risky, as measured by hospital admissions, than travel by car at any time of the year. The authors call for safer traffic environments, separating cyclists from car drivers where possible.

RTCs do not simply affect the car driver or passengers involved in a crash, nor the cyclist or pedestrian hit by a car. If any of these are killed there is a family (or families) left bereaved. In an interesting paper Sullivan and colleagues (2009) have sought to estimate the number of people in England and Wales who have lost a close family member due to a fatal RTC. Using the Longitudinal Study, which links individual records to Census data for all people born on four specific days of the year, they found that there were (between 1971 and 2005) 1801 deaths from RTCs, leaving just under 6500 close family members bereaved. Extending this to the population as a whole this suggests that almost 600,000 people would have been bereaved during this 34 year period. The financial and emotional cost of this suggests that the scale of the public health problem of RTCs needs to be recognised; there are huge indirect as well as direct consequences.

I want now to say something about policies that may help reduce the burden of RTCs. Driving requires concentration – hence the warning signs on British and other motorways encouraging drivers to 'take a break'. A high degree of cognitive functioning is needed, and there are penalties for those whose functioning is impaired through alcohol or drugs. Inevitably, perhaps, there are always drivers who should not be on the roads at any one point in time.

Concentration is impaired by mobile phone use, and this is now illegal in the UK while driving, though personal observation suggests the law is frequently flouted. Many other countries have similar legislation, though it varies by state/province in the USA and Canada. Evidence from Perth in Western Australia (McEvoy et al. 2005) suggests a driver using a mobile phone is four times as likely to have a car crash resulting in hospital attendance. In addition, those using hands-free devices also seem to be at risk. Those using a mobile phone are less aware of what is happening on the road, may fail to observe road signs, and have longer reaction times. Drivers who cover long distances (such as those driving a company car) are more likely than most to use a mobile phone while driving. While most drivers disapprove of this behaviour, about one-quarter admit to doing so.

As Tranter (2010) and others have pointed out, a simple reduction in speed is effective in reducing the risk of deaths to pedestrians; that risk is 85% if the car is travelling at 40 mph and remains high (45%) at 30 mph (the legal limit in most built-up areas of Britain); but it reduces to 5% if the car is travelling at 20 mph. There is good evidence that reducing traffic speed in urban areas reduces injuries from RTCs. Grundy and his colleagues (2009) have demonstrated the considerable benefits to public health from implementing 20 mph traffic speed zones in London. Since 1995 several cities in the UK have experimented with 20 mph zones and these are now quite common in London. Grundy and his team looked at casualty rates on detailed road segments before and after such zones were introduced. They demonstrate that casualties as a whole were reduced by 41%, the number of children killed or seriously injured was halved, and injuries to pedestrians were reduced by one-third. This is extraordinarily compelling evidence in favour of a wider introduction of such schemes, or a nationwide lowering of the speed limit. Work elsewhere in Europe suggests similar benefits. Tranter (2010) reports a study in Graz, Austria which demonstrated a 25% cut in serious road casualties when the speed limit was reduced to 30 kph (about 18 mph). As he notes, only half the residents surveyed before the limit was introduced supported the reduction, but this rose to 80% after the benefits were publicised.

Given the considerable use of both fixed and mobile speed cameras in the global north it is important to ask what impact these have on reducing injury and mortality on roads. Pilkington and Kinra (2005) undertook a systematic review of the literature and of 14 observational studies (mostly before and after installation studies) all but one showed that cameras were effective up to three years or less after their introduction. Reductions in outcomes ranged from 17% to 71% for deaths in the immediate vicinity of camera sites. Wilson and colleagues (2006) considered a set of studies that reported pre/post installation reductions in all crashes, including those with injuries. In the vicinity of camera sites these reductions ranged from 8% to 46% for injury crashes, and 40% to 45% for crashes that resulted in fatalities or serious injuries. Studies of the longer-term effects of such installation reveal that these improvements are maintained over time. In a study of rural Norfolk, UK, Jones and his colleagues (2008) compared injury statistics near 29 mobile camera sites with those in the rest of the county. Examining data for the two years before and after the introduction of speed cameras, they found that the number of vehicle crashes declined by 1% and crashes involving fatalities or serious injuries declined by 9% on the roads without cameras. However, at the camera sites, crashes were observed to decline by 19% and fatal and serious crashes by 44%. All this evidence suggests that such mobile cameras have a measurable benefit in reducing RTC incidence.

Adams (1995) has, with others, argued consistently that legislation to enforce the wearing of seat belts has simply served to transfer the risk from car drivers and passengers onto cyclists and pedestrians. The argument of this so-called 'risk compensation' hypothesis is that motorists feel safer as a result and this leads to a decline in the standard of driving; less awareness of others on or near the road. The same argument extends to bicycle helmets; cyclists may feel safer and take more risks on the road, while drivers may take less care if they see a helmeted cyclist. There are often quite polarised debates between those who consider that safety measures are the individual's responsibility (driver – buckle up; cyclist – wear your helmet) and those who argue that safety measures should be focused more on the traffic environment (speed traps, traffic calming, cycle lanes, improved lighting and so on). Unsurprisingly, road lighting has been shown to lessen the risk of road accident injury; research in Holland (Wanvik 2009) indicates that lighting lessens the risk of injury to pedestrian and cyclists, more so than for car and motorcycle users. While darkness increases the risk of accidents, the risk increases by 17% on lit rural roads and 145% on unlit roads.

Jacobsen and colleagues (2009) ask 'who owns the roads?' There is a subset of the population for whom this is a very pertinent question; the disabled 'other', particularly those who find it difficult or impossible to walk. Such individuals suffer a particular diminution of network capital and find themselves subject to inequalities of access that those without physical impairments do not necessarily experience. The built environment, around which many navigate unaided, can serve to exclude disabled people, adding to the discrimination they experience in other contexts. For example, pavements (sidewalks) in a poor state of repair, the 'clutter' of street furniture, poorly designed entrances to buildings, and signage that may be illegible or poorly positioned, all serve to exclude this othered group from mainstream society.

In the same way that walkers criticise the 'cultural hegemony' of the car driver, the disability writer and activist Mike Oliver (cited in Freund and Martin 2004: 283) has criticised the ways in which able-bodied people treat wheelchair users as 'other'. Urban design has, he argues, privileged the walker in a form of what he calls 'walkism'. The distinct benefits of walking do not extend to the wheelchair user having to negotiate unfriendly or poorly-designed streets. Nor do they always extend to the wheelchair user who wants easy access to shops and services lining those streets. While planners might complain about the costs of introducing more disability-friendly features into their designs Oliver draws attention to the massive investment in the air travel that provides 'mobility aids' for all those who are physically incapable of unaided flight! In recent years there has been improved access to public transport – required by legislation – for those with impairments. For example, low-floor buses, automated voice and screen information serve to improve travel possibilities.

Where does the responsibility for such access lie? Is it a matter of continually providing technological improvements to devices that might improve the mobility of the user? Or, should we be better at designing environments that improve access? In the UK, some disabled people in receipt of government-funded mobility allowances, can, via the charity 'Motability' lease a car, powered wheelchair or scooter. These go some way towards countering the 'social oppression' recognised by Gleeson (1999: 138). For him, restricted mobility inhibits the acquisition of social (network) capital as well as chances of gaining (and then getting to) meaningful employment. This in turn leads to a diminution in material resources and a perpetuation of social inequalities.

Stuck in the car

In the previous chapter I indicated the likely exposures to air pollution of those living on, or walking along, the streets down which motor vehicles travel. Car (automobile) drivers are exposed to different types of organic hydrocarbons, including inside the vehicle itself; evidence suggests that benzene is the most problematic of these organics (Schupp et al. 2006). While not concerned directly with drivers, an Indian study of petrol pump attendants and automobile service station workers in Kolkata (Calcutta) revealed high levels of benzene exposure from vehicular sources, and the exposed subjects had significantly more haematological and immunological alterations than matched controls (Ray et al. 2007). Research suggests that taxi drivers may be exposed to high levels of pollution. A study of Parisian taxi drivers revealed that concentrations of pollutants in their vehicles were considerably higher than in ambient Paris air and were similar to, or slightly above, the concentrations measured at fixed road-side sites (Zagury et al. 2000). Pollution risk increases with speed. Cars will produce 10-120% more CO_2 if travelling at 70 mph instead of 60 mph (Tranter 2010). Acceleration and braking increase pollution.

Drivers face other risks from what they inhale on the road. Wallensten et al. (2010) referred to evidence suggesting that drivers (particularly those driving as part of their job) are at increased risk of Legionnaires' disease; specifically, a five-fold increase in risk compared with other workers. This is because driving, or being a passenger in, a car that did not contain screen-wash in the windscreen wiper fluid is a health risk; the odds of getting the disease were almost 50 times greater than those in cars which did use screen-wash. The authors suggest that up to 20% of the sporadic cases of Legionnaires' disease might be prevented by using screen-wash – clearly, a cheap and effective public health intervention that would lead to fewer cases and fewer deaths. They also refer to *Legionella* (the bacterium) being isolated in rain puddles on the road, implying that there is a possible route of exposure via the aerosols inhaled as cars drive along the road.

In addition to impacts on respiratory health there are also impacts from road traffic noise, both in the global south and north. A spatial analysis of road traffic noise in Karachi, Pakistan (Mehdi et al. 2011) found that the average noise level across the city was over 66 decibels and peak levels were over 100 decibels, not far from the level thought to cause hearing impairment. A Swiss study of over 5000 adults (Dratva et al. 2010) found that 13% reported high annoyance from the noise of road traffic, and a significant inverse association with quality of life measures. More seriously, sleep can be disturbed, and there may be longer-term health effects, including raised blood pressure. These effects will inevitably be socially and geographically patterned, according to place of residence.

Motoring for many hours during the week is not good for musculoskeletal health and posture. While the vehicle is mobile the driver and her passengers are, in a very real sense, *im*mobile. Alvord, cited in Freund and Martin (2004: 278) suggests that rather 'than being ergonomically designed, car seats are fashioned to be comfortable for 8.5 minutes, the average time a customer sits in a seat when selecting a new car'!

Putnam (2000) has argued that lengthy commuting distances have led to the erosion of social capital. The majority of car commuting is undertaken by the driver alone (Urry 2002: 263) and, as the separation of home and workplace continues, the time left for social interaction and engagement in community life is reduced. As

Urry (2002: 264) observes, the physical separation of work, leisure, retail and home places requires extensive car travel to get from one place to the other. In rural areas the production and reproduction of social capital will often demand that people travel by car to meet for social and other interactions. Social participation of necessity requires movement from place to place and those left without access to a car or other form of transport may find themselves isolated and facing social exclusion.

There are also dis-benefits that will impact on mental health as a result of experiencing congestion, lengthy journeys to work and possible missed appointments. Those employed as drivers are also affected, especially when they are marginalised in society. For example, immigrant taxi drivers in Toronto find themselves subject to racist abuse and assault (both symbolic and actual violence), as well as economic uncertainty and exploitation by taxi firms (Facey 2008). Lack of job control, and competition among firms and drivers, can cause stress. At the extreme this translates into violent behaviour; in West Cumbria (NW England) a disaffected taxi driver killed 12 people in June 2010, including another taxi driver against whom a grudge regarding pick-ups (fares) was apparently lodged (http://news.bbc.co.uk/1/hi/england/10222188.stm).

A further 'risk' we can add to this list is so-called 'road rage', where drivers (over)react, occasionally with tragic consequences, to a real or imagined slight from other drivers or road users. Moran (2009: 93) cites the case of a 'previously blameless bus driver who was forced to brake suddenly by a Saab driver and then chased him for five miles through the streets of Bristol, while the bus's passengers were flung from their seats and screamed in terror'. While most of us have probably cursed – silently or loudly – what we consider to be poor behaviour on the road Moran suggests we are all susceptible to extreme reactions, since the road is 'a kind of parallel universe' where anyone was 'capable of undergoing a terrifying psychological transformation'. Road rage – a perceived invasion of personal space – does not just affect 'the maniacs and psychotics'; it is 'the dark heart of our inner selves' (Moran 2009: 93).

Laurier (2004) has conducted ethnographic research among car drivers which reveals that some of them undertake office work while mobile. As reported by Adey (2010: 180-1) the activities 'included continual communication with the office by dictating letters to distant secretaries, returning calls to complaining clients, reading and shuffling between different paper documents, *all while attempting to drive at the same time*' (my italics). The risks to the driver, passenger, and other road user are not remarked upon directly though Laurier does acknowledge that they 'sit for too long, get stuck in traffic jams, make mobile phone calls when they should not and break the legal speed limit to arrive at meetings on time' (Laurier 2004: 263).

Busin' an' truckin'

Stradling and his colleagues (2007) examine, in a Scottish context, what makes for a pleasant bus journey (and therefore might persuade people out of their cars). For some respondents there are the contemplative possibilities – the ability to 'switch off' and let the responsibility for the journey lie in the hands of the driver. There is time to read, reflect, and relax (Guiver 2007). Social bonds – albeit in general short in duration – get formed as people queue (stand in line) for the bus. Bus drivers can help. As one of Guiver's respondents in northern England puts it: 'it's a wonderful way of meeting people. I can have some really good laughs with some of the people on that bus and some of the drivers have got a wonderful sense of humour and you might be feeling wet, miserable, down but you get on that bus and somebody says "hello" to you it makes you feel a lot better. I mean there's a good community out there that use the bus routes and, I mean, I think that is lovely' (Guiver 2007: 238).

In some countries many of the fatalities among motorised vehicles are due to travelling on public buses and trucks; Naci and colleagues (2009) suggest that 26% of road traffic deaths in Russia are those travelling in buses and trucks, a figure rising to 32% in Ghana. They attribute this to the poor maintenance of vehicles, poor training of drivers and the overloading of such vehicles to maximise profit.

What is known about the health risks faced in their mobile workplaces by bus and truck (lorry) drivers? Evidence suggests there are risks of exposure to toxic substances in the driver's cabin and possible risks from remaining in a sitting position during the long-distance journeys made by truck drivers. Garshick and others (2008) obtained detailed work records for over 30,000 US truck drivers who were employed in 1985, and studied the risk of death from lung cancer between 1985 and 2000. Lung cancer mortality was associated with length of exposure (years worked in jobs associated with vehicle exhaust emissions). Such jobs included those involving driving in urban areas and along inter-city highways. One difficulty with this kind of study is in controlling for smoking rates (since these are known to be very significantly associated with lung cancer); the authors attempted this kind of adjustment, which slightly attenuated the effect of emissions exposure. Such exposure seemed to come as much from other vehicles and background air pollution as from within the driver's own vehicle. Regardless, exposure to diesel exhaust was deemed to be positively associated with lung cancer risk.

Drawing on a meta-analysis of epidemiological studies conducted on bladder cancer, there is evidence of a modest, but statistically significant increased risk of such cancer among bus drivers (Reulen et al. 2008). This could be due to exposure to diesel emissions. Again, studies need to control for other risk factors such as smoking (since the toxic substances – arylamines – from cigarette smoke can accumulate in urine and come into contact with the bladder lining) or, indeed, exposure to toxic chemicals in other environments.

Several studies of bus and truck drivers in Denmark point to serious health problems. Jensen and colleagues (2008) found significantly elevated risks of locomotor disease (including spinal disorders such as disc problems, shoulder, arm and back problems). These problems affected bus, long-haul and other truck drivers. Tüchsen and colleagues (2006) examined the risk of stroke among over 35,000 such drivers, finding that such groups were up to 50% more at risk than economically active men in Denmark as a whole. Other research they cite confirms similar findings for ischaemic heart disease. The possible explanations include psychosocial stress from working conditions (shift and night work, long driving hours in sedentary positions), leading to elevated blood pressure.

Quinn and her colleagues (2007) paint a graphic picture of the burden of occupational exposures encountered by school bus drivers (among other groups) in Boston. The diesel engines require a lengthy warm-up period before being driven, and as a result diesel exhaust lingers and soot accumulates, exposing bus drivers to dust and chemicals. On most routes, noise levels are high, whether due to bus engines, fractious children, or traffic. Psychosocial job strain results from poor passenger behaviour, dense city traffic, and difficulties in meeting time schedules (Quinn et al. 2007).

But not only bus drivers are exposed to air pollution; passengers are too. Some studies have looked at the exposures of children commuting to school by bus and have asserted that, because of sometimes lengthy journeys, these exposures can be considerable. Behrentz and colleagues (2005) measured fine particulate concentrations (also polycyclic aromatic hydrocarbons and benzene) in diesel-powered school buses in Los Angeles, finding that mean concentrations during the journey were between 20 and 40 times greater than while at the bus stop, these exposures being exacerbated when buses were travelling in a convoy with windows open or even when windows were closed and exhaust gases found their way into the bus.

Much of the literature focuses on environmental exposures to air pollution. But bus drivers face other risks. Possible stressors include poor vehicle (cabin) design, traffic congestion, threat of violence, and poor passenger behaviour, as well as organisational ones resulting from shift patterns and rest breaks (Tse et al. (2006). While the impact of these can be mediated by personality and gender, possible outcomes are cardiovascular disease and musculoskeletal problems, mental health concerns (anxiety and depression) and the work-related impacts (sickness absence and staff turnover). There are, of course, compensators for work-related stressors; for example, friendly and polite passengers and other road users who show consideration and courtesy to drivers mitigate the negative impacts highlighted here.

Much of the above research is cast in a classically epidemiological mould and has little to say about the lived experiences of travellers in cars and buses, particularly experiences which are not positive. Guiver (2007) used discourse analysis to explore how people talk about bus and car travel in cities in northern England. She identifies concerns about safety and vulnerability, and the quality of the journey. Some drivers are unhelpful, driving off before passengers are seated and ignoring 'loutish' behaviour by some younger travellers. Some buses are over-crowded. As she puts it, 'the worst-case scenarios focussed on the physical experience of using buses, especially the intrusion of other people (through smells, intimidation, litter, dirt, close proximity, fears for safety) appearing to induce a sense of violation of integrity' (Guiver 2007: 237). Stradling's work in Edinburgh, Scotland, confirms this, with fellow travellers variously described as intimidating, frightening and abusive (Stradling et al. 2007). Moreover, it is not simply the journey itself that may be problematic for the passenger. Waiting for a bus late at night carries risks if there are few other people about and the bus stop is not well lit.

Turning to truck (lorry) drivers, Handsley (2009) offers an account (sadly, all too brief) of his own experiences as a truck driver (before entering academia as a professional sociologist). While he has little to say about health as such, he does allude to both the feelings of camaraderie among fellow truckers, some of which is 'banter' exchanged on the airwaves or at truck stops, often involving conversations relating to, and demeaning of, women. But feelings of boredom are prevalent: 'much of the time, the trucker's life contained nothing more exciting than gazing at the rear of the truck in front'.

Truck (lorry) drivers in the global south have long been associated with the spread of HIV and other sexually transmitted infections, as evidence from countries in East Africa and in Brazil and India has suggested. Mobile populations such as these encounter situations that expose them to increased health risks, such as sexually transmitted infections (Lippman et al. (2007). There are more opportunities to engage in casual sex while working away from home, as there are fewer perceived constraints requiring these mobile workers to follow traditional norms and obligations. Lippman and her colleagues (2007) suggest that this high degree of mobility puts truckers into a 'liminal' space, one that engenders a sense of 'between-ness' that leads to risk-taking behaviour. Surveys of 1775 truck drivers crossing the Brazilian border in 2003 found that over one-quarter reported concurrent sexual partnerships and only 9% reported consistent condom use with their principal partner. Length of time spent on the road was associated with an increase in the likelihood of having commercial sex partners. But it is not only physical mobility that is associated with risky behaviours; it is also the extent to which truckers understood themselves to be in a liminal state (a greater perceived sense of freedom). As Lippman et al. (2007: 2471) have it, 'while norms value monogamy, behaviour on the road was indicative of increased freedoms, as if truckers got carried away by the environment'.

Concluding remarks

I have, in this chapter and elsewhere, made reference to Moran's engaging cultural history of the road (2009). But Moran has relatively little to say about the road as a risky environment; he says nothing (apart from one brief aside, 238 pages into his book) about the negative impact that roads have on those living on them – in terms of the burden of environmental pollution. Overall, he paints a fairly affectionate view of roads, which 'can be ruinous, but they are not a concrete napalm that renders all human life around them unbearable' (Moran 2009: 239). It cannot be denied that motor vehicles provide a lifeline for many. The car is an essential mode of transport for the rural dweller, while lorries/trucks provide the flexibility that train schedules cannot, and buses can provide a safe and convenient mode of transport for many.

In contrast, for others the car has, in large parts of the world, become almost the 'default setting' for journeys. In the global north we move through the world 'in motor-driven "wheel chairs" or sitting still at our computers' (Bergmann 2008a: 12). Bergmann suggests that this greatly reduces the sensual experience. We risk losing our sense of connection to local and natural surroundings because of this mode of travel. Further, set against the undeniable benefits of motor vehicles are considerable social costs, particularly of 'accidents' (and therefore injury and death) and of environmental damage. The burden of mortality and morbidity from road traffic crashes is a huge and unacceptable one, across the globe. I return to the environmental consequences in a concluding chapter, where I consider briefly the links between mobilities and climate change.

Chapter 4
Trains, and Boats and Planes

Introduction

As with road travel, the movements of people and goods by rail, ship and air, are intertwined with material infrastructure that is itself immobile. Railway stations and tracks, ports and their docks, airports and check-in desks: all these are things that facilitate movement but are not themselves mobile. The mobilities literature in cultural sociology makes much of this. Here, I focus attention on three modes of mobility – the train, the boat/ship, and the airplane – and their health impacts.

I first examine some health dimensions of train travel, looking at both the health benefits and some of the negative aspects (such as accidents and the opportunities presented to those seeking to end their life). Turning to those travelling on water there are, as with rail travel, risks to those enabling the mobilities of others as well as both benefits and risks in travelling on cruise ships, for example. The last section focuses on air travel. As Urry (2007: 153) observes, air transport 'makes possible very many different mobilities, of holidaymaking, money laundering, business travel, the drug trade, infections, international crime, asylum seeking, leisure travel, arms trading, people smuggling and slave trading'. I shall examine in another chapter the ways in which air traffic can expedite the transmission of disease across the globe but focus my attention here on the direct health impacts on people who travel by air. Some attention is also given to those not themselves travelling but who are exposed to health risks by virtue of their living close to airports.

Letting the train take the strain

The development of the rail network in the nineteenth century transformed travel and the way in which travellers engaged with place and landscape. But this engagement took time; initially, railways 'were hated destroyers of natural landscapes, and the crooked cabals that brought them into being make today's road lobbyists seem like benevolent amateurs' (Moran 2009: 251). They also changed people's perception of movement: 'As velocity dissolved the foreground, train travellers felt as if they no longer belonged to the same space as the perceived objects which passed by so quickly' (Aitchison et al. 2000: 40). For some this was stimulating, but for others less so; the sensation of speed terrified some travellers (Bissell 2008: 57). And these experiences have to be set against those of some (in both the 19th and 20th centuries: see Stevenson, 2009 on Victorian women rail travellers) whose journeys in enclosed compartments (compared with today's open ones) exposed them to threats from fellow travellers (Bissell 2008: 51).

Rail journeys for business or pleasure are much more common in Europe than in North America. Urry (2007: 107) reports on a study of 25,000 rail passengers in the UK which found – not altogether surprisingly – that those travelling on business were likely to be working on the train while leisure travellers were more likely to be gazing at the passing landscapes, reading for pleasure, or observing others around them. Most business travellers found that the travel time was not wasted (though substantial delays are clearly likely to be stressful). As Urry notes, one major UK rail company (Virgin) has advertised its trains as providers of valuable thinking time!

Bissell (2009b) conducted an ethnographic study of 46 long-distance railway passengers travelling between Edinburgh and London. His focus is on the sociality of the journey but there are some suggestions of relationships to well-being. For example, a lone female traveller complains about feeling vulnerable on the platform in the absence of many station staff. Sexual harassment is sometimes encountered. In India the problem has been so serious that women-only train services, known as 'Ladies Specials', are operated in the major cities.

Bissell also describes the strategies that passengers use to protect their personal space, such as the placement of luggage on seats and belongings on tables. Passengers can find it quite stressful if they cannot keep sight of valuable cases. Any slights or resentments (for example, from loud or disruptive passengers) are felt more directly than in cars, where the window or windscreen can insulate the driver from someone s/he may have offended. Delays, if serious, can 'bring about different forms of collectivity whilst on the move where the solitary enclosures that passengers forge are momentarily broken down' (Bissell 2009b: 61). But when the train does arrive these little bonds and courtesies may disappear in the scramble for seats. Bissell, though, stresses the positive aspects, asserting that simple social interactions add to the pleasure of the journey. Elsewhere (Bissell 2008) he looks at the visual experience of the journey, noting how this is affected by the material construction of the railway compartment. For example, whether one sits facing the direction of travel or facing backwards gives one a different journey experience (as well as inducing nausea among some who face backwards). And one's batteries can be recharged, so to speak, from particular journeys. 'Whilst one-off tourist travellers might be enchanted by the mesmeric capacities of the passing landscape, weary commuters and contemplative business travellers may be equally susceptible. Indeed for them, disengaged, sublime vision has the capacity to soothe and recharge the body' (Bissell 2008: 48).

For older adults journeys can be liberating, as Levin (2009) has documented in Sweden. Some of her respondents, all over 70 years of age, travel 100 km or more, by public transport, to visit friends regularly, extending this to up to 500 km during weekends, Levin suggests these trips are invaluable for their well-being and maintaining their confidence and social skills; the memories and stories of their trips are very important. One woman traveller travelled by train every day to and from home, knitting and chatting to people because she did not want to be alone at home (Levin 2009: 151). This work is an important counter to the dominant mobility discourses of the younger adult (car/plane) traveller and suggests that not all older adults' mobilities are impaired or stressful.

What are the negative impacts of rail travel on mental health? Little is known about the stresses of commuting by rail. Evans and Wener (2006) looked at a sample of suburban rail 208 commuters (both men and women) travelling to and from New York City. The longer the journey, the higher were levels of perceived stress. The authors argue that commuting stress is an important and neglected form of environmental health. Delays to journeys can create stress, and (as with other forms of transport) it is tempting – though usually unfair – to blame the visible guard or attendant when s/he may have played no part at all in the factor/s causing the delay. Equally, those used to rail travel in Britain will probably have experienced over-crowding and the occupancy of one's reserved seat by another passenger who may react inappropriately to a request to move – thereby causing stress to both parties and perhaps to any onlookers. Further, there are real concerns about safety, as when Budd (2009) expresses nervousness about bus travel shortly after the London bombings in July 2005. Rail travellers have expressed similar concerns. One of Bissell's respondents admitted that: 'I know it's really daft but after the attacks in London you know if you see a young Muslim guy with a beard and a rucksack, you do feel a bit uneasy about sitting in the same carriage as him' (quoted in Bissell 2008: 51).

In the early 1990s the rail system in Britain was reorganised. The state-run British Rail, which had operated both the train service and the infrastructure (stations and rail track) was split into two components. The infrastructure became the provenance of a new company, Railtrack (now Network Rail), while the train routes were divided among different organisations. Between 1996 and 2003 there were several high-profile accidents and accompanying fatalities, leading some to claim that privatisation had worsened safety on the rail network. Evans (2007) has looked at time series data on rail accidents in Britain between 1967 and 2003 to determine whether safety has worsened as a result of rail privatisation. The evidence suggests that accident rates were declining well before privatisation in 1993 (Figure 4.1). Indeed, data from as far back as 1945 confirm that there has been a gradual, non-linear decline in accident rates well into the 21st century. Evans suggests that high-profile, and clearly serious, accidents are easily recalled, leading people to over-estimate the probability of major incidents and fatalities.

Some rail accidents involve releases of toxic chemicals. In the US a system exists for collecting data on such releases (the Hazardous Substances Emergency Events Surveillance system) and this revealed that, between 1999 and 2004 about 9% of all reports (1165 events) involved rail accidents. Some of these were serious; for example, in South Carolina the collision in January 2005 of a freight train carrying chlorine released 11,500 gallons of chlorine gas, killing nine people and causing organ damage to over 500 others (MMWR, 2005). A state of emergency was declared and almost 5500 residents evacuated. Given that there

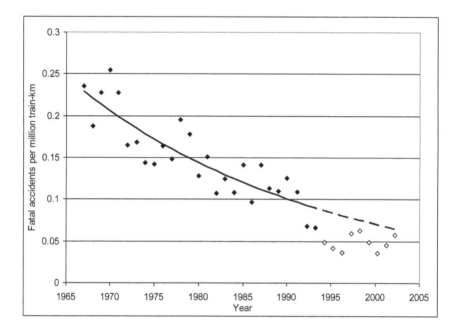

Figure 4.1   Fatal rail accidents in Britain, 1967-2003

Source: Reprinted with permission from Evans (2007): 516.

are over 4000 rail shipments of very hazardous materials each day across the US, travelling through densely populated areas, there are clear risks to the health of local residents and rail employees.

I looked in some detail in the last chapter at exposure to air pollution from pedestrian and road travel. It might be imagined that exposures from rail travel would be minimal. However, on subway systems this appears not to be entirely the case. A small study of personal exposures of office workers to airborne manganese in London showed that mean exposure was relatively high, due to the fact that some commuted via the underground railway system where airborne dust and metal concentrations are ten times higher than those in the general environment (Pfeifer et al. 1999). There are several possible sources for this, including brake wear and mechanical wear of train wheels on the steel rails. A German study (Fromme et al. 1998) found high levels of polycyclic aromatic hydrocarbons in the passenger compartment of a subway train, possibly due to the use of wood preservatives on wooden railway ties. Laden et al. (2006) have shown an elevated risk of lung cancer mortality in over 52,000 US railroad workers exposed to diesel exhaust. Among workers hired after 1945, when diesel locomotives were first introduced, the relative risk of lung cancer was 1.77 and there was evidence that risk increased with length of exposure. Workers hired before 1945 had a lower relative risk (1.30) and in that group there was no evidence of a dose response with duration of exposure. This study has proved controversial, in part because one needs to control for other variables that affect lung cancer (most obviously smoking).

Historically, the development of the railroad in the second half of the nineteenth century in the US provided the conditions for the emergence of new forms of mobilities, namely vagrants using the railroad for travel. Anderson (1961: 87) distinguishes three types of vagrant: the hobo, the tramp and the 'bum'. 'The hobo works and wanders, the tramp dreams and wanders and the bum drinks and wanders'. A hobo is a homeless person who travels in search of work. The first hobos were those employed to work on the construction of the American railroads in the second half of the nineteenth century, but they became 'the in-between worker, willing to go anywhere to take a job and equally willing to move on later' (Anderson 1961: xviii). The city (and Chicago was *the* city for the hobo) was the place to secure a new job elsewhere in the country, but it was also a place for medical attention. 'For the sick and injured of the floating fraternity Chicago is a haven of refuge because of the large number of opportunities found here for free treatment' (Anderson 1961: 13). Hobos actively sought new situations, new places and new journeys, but as automobile travel took off the hobo disappeared.

Anderson's book is less about the hobo's journey and more about their experiences in the city. But he does have a little to say about the health of the hobo (and homeless men in general). He reports on a study of 400 hobos riding freight trains from Salt Lake City, Utah, to Chicago in the summer of 1921 (Anderson, 1961: 127). He noted 50 'defects' among 48 persons, including serious eye problems, various injuries and impairments, and what we would now call learning disabilities. He also refers to their (ill)health at work, due to exposure to temperature extremes and to accidents. Others argued that the health problems suffered by tramps and hobos were inherited conditions and that even the desire to wander (wanderlust or 'dromomania') was inherited (Cresswell 2001: 115-6). Tramps and hobos were also blamed for the spread of sexually transmitted disease. The incidence of syphilis was linked to migrant workers and helped in the portrayal of the tramp as a dangerous person. The tramp embodied deviance, and disease. Anderson also comments on the risks faced by the railroad hobo. His data suggest that, in 1919, 2553 'trespassers' (not necessarily all hobos) were killed on the rail lines, and 2658 were injured (Anderson 1961: 161). Not everyone regretted such deaths. The editor of the St Louis Journal in 1879 noted that 'a wrecked freight car invariably means a dead tramp', and these provide 'an expensive but effective way of getting rid of a very undesirable class of nuisances' (cited in Cresswell 2001: 10).

The railway also provides an opportunity for some seriously disturbed or distressed people to commit suicide. Evidence suggests that the railway accounts for between 3-7% of all suicides (compared with the more common means of poisoning, drowning of hanging). What do we know about the descriptive epidemiology of railway suicide? I consider this with reference to the railway system in England and Wales – including the London Underground (subway system) – and in Germany.

Clarke (1994) looked at data over a 100-year period (1850-1949) in England and Wales. The number of railway suicides increased steadily during the first 60 years, with about 200 male deaths and 180 female deaths in 1910. The numbers dropped dramatically during the First World War but rose to well over 200 for both men and women, before dropping again between 1939 and 1945. To some extent the increases mirror both the growth of rail track and the volume of rail traffic. Clarke's study showed that railway suicide is more common among younger adults than is true of suicide in general, and that males were more likely to choose this method. In the former West Germany, Schmidtke (1994) looked at more recent data (1976-84). Of over 6000 such suicides, the ratio of males to females was 2.54 to 1. Among men, over a quarter were in the 20-29 year age bracket; the age profile among women was more even, but railway suicide was more common among older women (in their late 50s). Schmidtke also looked at temporal variability. There were significant excess suicides for men in October, while women seemed more likely to commit suicide in December and January. Both men and women were more likely to take their lives on Mondays and Tuesdays, possibly because the rest of the week 'lies ahead of them like a mountain' (Schmidtke 1994: 424). Men were more likely to commit suicide in the evening (18.00-21.00) and while women also chose this time-frame they were as likely to commit suicide in the afternoon.

Schmidtke finds some evidence of temporal clustering in railway suicides, which could be explained as an 'imitation' effect. Following a German television series on the suicide of a young male student there was a significant increase in suicides among 15-29 year old males (62 deaths in the 70 days following the screening, compared with only 33 during an average 70 day period). Baumert and colleagues (2005) have updated Schmidtke's study, looking at the (unified) Germany between 1991 and 2000. There were, on average, 17 suicides each week on German railways; a not inconsiderable public health problem. As other studies have shown, the incidence is higher among younger adults and the pattern was for the incidence among young people to increase over time. In addition, such people were choosing open tracks, rather than railway stations, as the location.

O'Donnell and Farmer (1994) have examined the epidemiology of suicide on the London Underground, while Clarke and Poyner (1994) have proposed some ideas to mitigate the risk. The average number of suicides increased from 36 a year in the 1940s to 94 in the 1980s, a much higher increase than observed on the mainline rail network. The incidence was significantly higher in March. Incidence was constant through the week, though markedly less on Sundays (when fewer trains tended to run). Over 40% of the incidents were between 10.00 and 16.00, and there was a significant gender bias (64% were men). As with other railway suicides, the peak age group for men is 25-34, though for women it is more evenly distributed by age group. Interestingly, there is significant geographical clustering; after adjusting for the differing traffic volumes at stations, there were significantly more suicides at stations with psychiatric hospitals close by. It appeared that those involved were often receiving treatment at such hospitals.

These extreme forms of mobility practices generate a significant burden. The mobilities of other travellers get seriously disrupted as lines are closed for investigations and recovery. Aside from the distress to families and friends, those directly involved (station staff, drivers, passengers) suffer from the experience. The emotional cost to the train driver is expressed in a short autobiographical account by Robert Hart (2009), one of whose colleagues was known as 'killer' because he had had seven suicides on his rail tracks. Hart himself had experienced two and expresses his feelings this way: 'I have tried to keep my distance: the more involved you get, the more emotional it all becomes. What angers me is why they want to involve a third person. They wanted to kill themselves, but I didn't want to kill them' (Hart 2009: 77-8).

What scope is there for the prevention of railway suicides? Suggestions (Clarke and Poyner 1994) include modifications to the station environment or to the trains. Thus, platform barriers, fitted with gates to allow access when the train stops, are one possibility. CCTV and improved staff training to spot potential victims can be employed. However, there must, sadly, be a limit to the effectiveness of interventions.

Plain sailing

Although the literature is much more sparse, some writers have looked at the health and well-being gains from travel by boat and ship. I should add that I refer here to those doing so by choice, and with the means to travel in some style. For example, in an interesting chapter Kleinert (2009) has undertaken ethnographic research on German-speaking, long-distance, long-term leisure cruisers, who rendezvous with others in New Zealand in preparation for ocean yacht travel that will take them over the globe. Although at sea there is physical isolation, modern communication technologies mean that complete isolation is a thing of the past. New and renewed social bonds form on dry land and in the harbours. This slow-paced (and very privileged) mobility contrasts with the 'hypermobilities' that we shall see in the next section. As Kleinert notes, it links mobility and dwelling, since for months at a time the yacht becomes a home: 'dwelling-in-motion' as she puts it (in much the same way as some people own house-boats moored along canals and rivers in the UK). It is not all 'plain sailing' however, since work has to be undertaken when things go wrong. So her respondents joke that 'cruising is fixing your boat in exotic places' (Kleinert 2009: 162). Overall, however, one can imagine that conjoining the economic capital that yacht owners have, with the network capital they enjoy, adds greatly to the health and well-being of this privileged group. Others travelling regularly and frequently by boat include those living on islands off the coast of British Columbia, Canada. For them ferry boats assist in the social organization and cultural life on these island communities (Vannini and Vannini 2009: 230). But the consequences for health and healthcare delivery have yet to be fully excavated.

While there has been considerable research on emissions from land-based mobile sources of pollution the impact of sea-borne sources has been neglected. Ship emissions are a significant component of global air pollution as they can be transported considerable distances as well as having local impacts on nearby coastal populations. Deniz and Durmusoglu (2008) quantified the considerable burden of emissions in the Sea of Marmara, Turkey (the body of water that links the Aegean to the Black Sea), which sees nearly 90,000 domestic and international vessels pass through each year. Some 20,000 tonnes of SO_2, and 87,000 tonnes of NO_x are estimated as annual emissions. Until recently the diesel exhaust emissions carried a high sulphur content but there are now stronger controls. In 1996 the US Environmental Protection Agency issued a requirement to US oil refineries to produce ultra-low-sulfur (sulphur) diesel fuel in order to substantially reduce emissions. They argued that the switch from high-sulphur fuel to low-sulphur fuel would prove an effective means of reducing particulate air emissions near land and would have a positive impact on public health in coastal areas. Their estimates were that fuel switching would improve public health by producing a 95% reduction in sulphur dioxide (SO_2) and an 85% reduction in fine particulate matter (PM). Winebrake and others (2009) suggest that these controls could reduce the number of premature deaths from all causes by over 40,000.

The large volume of ocean-going traffic, particularly that carrying oil supplies, generates a risk of oil spillage that sometimes transforms into major disasters. A good example is the Exxon Valdez oil spill in 1989 which released 40 million litres of crude oil onto the Alaskan coast, causing major ecological damage. There is evidence of serious mental health effects in local communities. Palinkas and colleagues (1993) surveyed 600 people 12 months after the spillage and found that the prevalence of generalised anxiety disorder was 20%; those persons with higher exposure to the disaster were 3.6 times as likely to show these symptoms as a control group. Women, and native Alaskans, were more at risk than others, leading the authors to conclude that the mental health consequences were as severe for some as the ecological impacts. It is too early to predict the long-term health consequences of the 2010 Deepwater Horizon oil spill in the Gulf of Mexico; but short-term respiratory symptoms and nausea were reported by those involved in cleaning up the oil, while concerns have been expressed about inhalation of potentially carcinogenic volatile organic compounds (both benzene in the oil and some of the concentrated chemical dispersants).

The expansion of travel aboard cruise ships and, to some extent, the growth of ferry traffic, has spawned new sets of risks (Cliff et al. 2009: 314-6). At least once a year the British press report on another outbreak of gastrointestinal illness that has resulted in a cruise ship's immobility, as opposed to the mobility that encourages people to undertake journeys to unfamiliar ports (and to undertake short trips when they reach such ports). Cramer and colleagues (2006) noted that the incidence of diarrhoeal disease on cruise ships declined from 29 cases per 100,000 passenger days in 1990 to only 16 in 2000. However, between 2001 and 2004 the incidence appeared to have increased again. Rooney and colleagues (2004) attribute the outbreaks to a wide range of pathogens, of which 'noroviruses' are common, as are species of *Salmonella*. The latter reflect poor temperature control in kitchens, contaminated raw ingredients and the cross-contamination of food (seafood is a particular problem). The spread of such disease can be contained by adequate cleaning of public rest-rooms (toilets) and other surfaces. But Neri and others (2008) note that some outbreaks caused by noroviruses are due to passengers who were unwell prior to boarding the ships. Whether, as they suggest, passengers could be adequately screened before embarkation seems a little impractical, but measures such as encouraging better hand-washing by passengers and crew and providing dispensers for hand sanitation are likely to be beneficial.

It is an interesting question whether disease outbreaks are the 'fault' of passengers and crew who do not engage in appropriate health behaviours (basic hygiene) or whether the owners and managers of cruise ships and ferries are failing to invest sufficiently in staff and other resources needed to maintain public health onboard such vessels. Certainly, other pathogens, such as *Legionella*, cannot be easily contained by the passengers and crew. The *Legionella* bacterium colonizes water distribution systems and air conditioning systems, as well as recreational pools and can therefore be assumed to be widespread on cruise ships and ferries. Azara et al. (2006) sampled water on board nine ships docked in Sardinia in 2004 and found that 42% of the water samples were contaminated by species of *Legionella*, with ferries particularly at risk. Goutziana and colleagues (2008) found no *Legionella* on cruise ships but three-quarters of ferries sampled in Greece tested positive; older ferries were particularly prone to show evidence of the bacterium, putting passengers and crew members at risk. Investment in improving infrastructure is clearly required.

In addition to crew on tour ships there are significant numbers working as fishermen and in merchant shipping, and both groups incur very significant health risks while mobile. Trawler fishing and merchant seafaring have long been the most hazardous of occupations. Roberts (2002) reports that between 1976 and 1995 fishermen were over 50 times more likely, and merchant seafarers 26 times more likely, to have a fatal accident at work than other British workers. These risks dwarf those of other occupations. In a more recent overview Oldenburg and his colleagues (2010) refer to significant occupational exposures to benzene and other carcinogens in engine rooms; and to ultraviolet (UV) radiation exposure from sunlight that may account for documented excess risks of lip and skin cancer. In addition, long absences from home result in isolation and stress, perhaps encouraging excess alcohol consumption; the incidence of depression and suicide is relatively high in this group too. The remoteness of the ship from centres of medical expertise creates problems of accessing care, though telehealthcare might obviate this if more widely used (see Chapter 11). Last, the risk of piracy cannot be ignored. Oldenburg and colleagues cite over 400 attempted or successful hijacks in 2009, especially in the South China Sea and off the east coast of Africa. In 2008 almost 800 crew members were reportedly taken hostage.

One major tragedy occurred close to the writer's home when, in February 2004, 21 Chinese workers drowned after being caught in an incoming tide in Morecambe Bay, North West England. They were so-called 'cockle pickers' who had been harvesting cockles (edible bivalves) but, having entered the country illegally under the control of a Chinese 'gangmaster', were unaware of the dangers of the work. Two forms of mobilities are at work here. First, the mobility that brings migrants from across the globe in search of work and, second, the local, poorly monitored mobility that saw their welfare appallingly neglected. See: www.guardian.co.uk/uk/2007/jun/20/ukcrime.humanrights, for an overview of this.

Up, up and away

The volume of passengers carried by air has grown hugely in recent years. Between 1952 and 2002, the number of terminal passengers at UK airports rose from 2.8 million to 188.8 million (Social Trends 2004, Vol. 34). US air carrier data (Bureau of Transportation Statistics) indicate that the number of passengers boarding international flights in the US rose from 5.7 million in July 1996 to 9.3 million in July 2010. The world's busiest airport (Atlanta) had a throughput of over 88 million passengers in 2009, up from 80 million in 2000; the number of passengers at Beijing international airport doubled from 27 million in 2002 to 55 million in 2009. As with other modes of transport, there are risks of accidents and – from serious accidents – death. But the numbers of accidents, and accompanying deaths, have dropped over the last 40 years. In 1970 there were 279 reported air accidents, but only 190 in 2000 (www.baaa-acro.com). The fatal accident rate in the 1990s was 1 per 700,000 flights, but only 1 for every 1.2 million flights during the first decade of the 21st century. Given the substantial growth in traffic these reductions are noteworthy. And it is of course worth contrasting the accident rate with that on the roads; 2220 people were killed on Britain's roads in 2009, three times as many as were killed *globally* in air accidents (*Guardian*, 5 January 2011: 6).

The literature on globalisation (and particularly, on world city networks) has placed considerable emphasis on studying the structure of global air travel. The expanding aeromobilities literature has plenty to say on the embodied experiences of air travel but is rather light on the health impacts. As I show in more detail in Chapter 9 we cannot begin to understand contemporary international disease spread without looking at how air travel networks serve to structure such diffusion

Issues of inequality were touched on in the first chapter. They are played out starkly in the airport setting, even though some literature on aeromobilities has tended to focus mostly on the global (usually male), well-networked, Western business traveller. As Crang (2002: 573) has it, the image of the airport as a networked space 'may speak to a globe-trotting semiotician, but says little to the family with overtired children delayed by a lack of connecting buses in Majorca'! There is, Cresswell (2006), shows, a kinetic hierarchy, with the frequent international flyer occupying a more privileged location in this space than the cleaner or baggage handler who comes from West Africa. Cresswell interviews those lower down the hierarchy, including dispossessed homeless people who use the airport for warmth, shelter, discarded food and reading matter. Providing such people are reasonably clean and decently dressed they are treated (at least at Schiphol, Amsterdam) no differently from the travellers sleeping for a few hours while awaiting a flight. Clearly, the same place offers a rich range of mobility experiences, ones that intersect but in truth represent very different worlds. As Crang (2002: 571) suggests, in the busy modern airport 'people pass but nobody meets'. Of course, it can be a very dangerous place, as in January 2011 at Domodedovo Airport (Moscow) when a suicide bomber caused death on a large scale.

In the early days of air travel, most was for business purposes and not for leisure. But this does not mean that such travellers were uninterested in the view below. Historical cultural studies of air travel tell us that when commercial air travel was a novelty, flying was generally regarded as an exciting adventure (Budd 2009) and airlines vied with each other to provide rich descriptions of the routes to 'incidental tourists' (Pirie 2009b). Frequent stop-overs meant that sightseeing on the ground became possible (for example, in the 1930s there were about 30 stops on the flight from London to Cape Town!). While many started out as incidental tourists most became 'captive' tourists (Pirie 2009b).

Most of the aeromobilities literature focuses on travel to and from international airports via major airlines. But, as van den Scott (2009: 211) puts it, 'not all that flies is fast or shines' and this leads her to examine regional air travel to and from a remote community (Arviat) in Nunavut, northern Canada. Here, citizens (mostly native Canadians) rely entirely on flights in order to get in and out of the town, including accessing hospital care. Cancellations and delays are inevitable and have consequences beyond mere inconvenience. Referring to a serious road incident that injured two girls one of van den Scott's respondents tells her that 'the plane couldn't land. It was foggy and everything. [The girls] were at the Health Centre with no doctor, with broken legs, broken arms and teeth sunk right in, um, for three, four days. Yeah, that's what happens when you can't get any plane' (van den Scott 2009: 217). But when the planes are flying strong social bonds emerge. These help them cope with the sense of alienation when travelling to the nearest major city (Winnipeg), over three hours away by air.

Considerable attention has been paid in recent years to the risks of deep vein thrombolysis (DVT) – also known as venous thromboembolism – among air travellers. In this condition, blood flow is restricted, ostensibly by the immobility of the traveller during flights. A review of 25 studies by Philbrick and colleagues (2007) suggested that the risk is indeed increased among those travelling for more than six hours and exacerbated among those at prior risk of DVT. Those in non-aisle seating, where passengers tend to be less mobile in-flight, are more at risk (Silverman and Gendreau 2009). For those who can afford the luxury of first-class or premium travel, where there is more leg-room and opportunity for movement, these risks might be lessened, suggesting a social (income) class gradient in risk.

However, an empirical study in New Zealand (Hughes et al. 2003) suggested that the risk applies to travellers of all classes.

Cabin pressure can be a health problem for some, particularly those with prior heart or respiratory conditions. Silverman and Gendreau (2009) studied volunteers exposed to a simulated 20 hour flight, who reported fatigue, light-headedness, headache and nausea that increased with increasing altitude and cabin pressure. The same symptoms (plus dry eyes, skin irritation, and stuffy noses) are associated with poor cabin air quality. Data on the frequency of serious medical incidents or emergencies are sparse, but Silverman and Gendreau (2009) note that US-registered airlines report 50-100 in-flight medical events every day, a figure that is comparable with that reported by British Airways. In order to deal with routine, and some serious, medical problems during flight commercial aircraft carry medical kits, including defibrillators, and there are links to sources of medical advice on the ground.

Exposure to cosmic radiation, even among frequent fliers, seems to be a minor risk, though pregnant cabin crew are advised to limit long-haul trips. Jet lag is a common, though relatively minor, problem for many international travellers, characterised by daytime fatigue, sleep-wake disturbances, decreased appetite and reduced coordination and cognitive skills (Silverman and Gendreau 2009). Travelling east causes difficulty in falling asleep because the body 'clock' has a natural tendency to resist shortening the daily cycle. Jet lag can be mitigated by simple therapies; a Cochrane review of 10 studies (clinical trials) suggested that taking between 0.5 and 5g of melatonin at the preferred bedtime at the destination could prevent or reduce jet lag (Silverman and Gendreau 2009).

In recent years considerable public attention has focused on air quality within commercial aircraft. This concerns the health of air crew in particular (there is a dearth of research on air quality within the body of aircraft). The background is that air is bled off from the engines and cooled before being piped inside the airplane; however, fumes from engine oil may leak into the air system and be therefore inhaled by crew and passengers. A UK Government Committee (the Committee on Toxicity) reviewed evidence on this in 2007 and suggested that an association between cabin air and pilot ill-health could not be proved or disproved. Since then studies are ongoing to sample cabin air for TCPs (tricresyl phosphates) that are known to be present in engine oils (as anti-wear agents). TCPs are organophosphates, and since the latter have been the focus of health concerns in other contexts, it is these chemicals that have been of primary interest when looking at the possibility of contaminated air. Pilots flying two types of aircraft in particular (BAe 146 and Boeing 757) have reported a 'distinctive and unpleasant oily, chemical smell' (Ross, 2008: 116) but apart from a small number of 'acute' incidents (news.bbc.co.uk/1/hi/uk/7053925.stm) these appear to be generally accepted as 'normal', and little formal reporting or recording seems to take place. In 2009, as part of an investigation by a German television network, ARD, and Schweizer Fernsehen (Swiss television), 31 swab samples were taken from the aircraft cabins of popular airlines; 28 were found to contain high levels of TCP (www.telegraph.co.uk/travel/travelnews/4610474/Toxic-cabin-air-found-in-new-plane-study.html).

Relatively little detailed research has been conducted on this so-called 'aerotoxic syndrome' and there is a need for well-designed epidemiological studies. These are likely to prove difficult, since the exposures are hard to quantify and tend to be short-term 'fume' events (occurring during take-off and landing, rather than throughout a flight). There is evidence (Ross 2008) that air contaminated by TCPs is neurotoxic, causing loss of balance, nausea, fatigue and 'cognitive impairment' (memory problems, reduced reaction times). Clearly, these are alarming, given the subjects of study. Campaign groups have emerged to represent the interests of air crew in this regard; for example, the Global Cabin Air Quality Executive (www.gcaqe.org) represents pilots, cabin crew and engineers and seeks to raise awareness of the issues. For passengers, a particular focus has been the diffusion of respiratory disease via re-circulated air within the aircraft. Fresh air is supplied from the plane's engines during the flight, but 50% of the air is re-circulated, partly to improve fuel efficiency. The re-circulated air passes through high efficiency particulate air filters (HEPAs) in order (in principle) to remove dust, bacteria and viral particles.

There are, of course, more subtle and less easily measurable health issues associated with air travel, whether engendered by flight delays, the discomfort of the journey itself, or the anxieties engendered among some during the flight (particularly during take-off and landing, but also when encountering periods of turbulence). Recently, publicity has been given to the scanning technologies that provide 'naked' images of passengers for the purposes of security screening, knowledge of which may also add to the stress of the air traveller.

Many worries about air travel may increase in the periods shortly after publicised aircraft crashes or terrorist attacks. The experience of waiting in long queues (lines) for check-in, and then often obtrusive security checks, is something that many find stressful, especially if accompanied by young children, older adults, or those with mobility difficulties. There are considerable inequalities in the lived experiences of different classes of travellers. This variation reflects differential access to air travel. Adey et al. (2007: 782) report on a study of travel from UK airports that suggested people in lower status social groups made 6% of all flights, while comprising 27% of the population. In turn, such groups were more likely to use low-cost 'hubs' (such as Stansted) and find themselves on low-cost airlines with relatively few cabin crew, tightly packed seats, and limited catering.

We should also consider the effects on those who travel regularly by air on business. Nynäs (2008), for example, has studied the diaries of those travelling to work at power plant construction sites for months at a time. He notes that while one project manager recalled a sense of excitement when travelling abroad early in his career, this has evaporated: 'Now, it is just waiting all the time, in airports, hotels and so on, and in between that there is nothing' (Nynäs 2008: 162). The sameness of the locations involved (airports, hotels, offices) adds to the sense of dislocation or inability to relate to a place.

Air travellers are also exposed, on relatively rare occasions, to the inconsiderate behaviour of other travellers, behaviour that may develop into 'air rage' if passengers have consumed excess alcohol. Of course, travellers also include cabin crew and on long-haul flights there are several of these, whose health and well-being can be affected by those with whom they are working, as well as the travelling public. They may be exposed to the same stressors as passengers. Whitelegg (2009) has examined the emotional labour undertaken by airline cabin crew (and such crew are still predominantly women), suggesting that this involves listening to, and being listened to by, fellow workers. While there is camaraderie in the shared experience of work, there is also emotional bonding and healing ('Jump-Seat Therapy') to be undertaken. As he notes, cabin crew are the ultimately mobile: one of his interviewees had travelled over ten million miles during her 21 years with (now-defunct) Pan Am.

Major international airports have become sites of commerce and entertainment, and are places that meet many needs of travellers. They are a powerful symbol of second modernity, signalling connectivity to global networks (Kesselring 2008). But this connectivity has other consequences. After the terrorist attacks on the twin towers on September 11th 2001 airports have become sites of surveillance and control, the experience of which intensified after the plot (using apparently innocuous bottled soft drinks) to blow up passenger aircraft mid-Atlantic in August 2006.

It would be remiss not to say more about the devastating impact of terrorist attacks that have used aircraft as the weapon. Considerable research effort has gone into understanding the longer-term consequences of the attack on the World Trade Center (WTC) in New York City, on September 11th 2001. While this (and the attack on the Pentagon and the crash in Pennsylvania) also killed passengers and left many bereaved, the main focus has been on examining: the health impacts on rescue workers; the mental health of those evacuated from the 'twin towers'; and the wider impacts on the mental health of those living in surrounding areas. Without attempting a comprehensive overview let me consider examples of each of these three impacts.

First, Aldrich and his colleagues (2010) have conducted a major study of the respiratory health of almost 13,000 fire department workers who attended the WTC in the aftermath; 343 workers had been killed. The collapse of the towers produced a dense dust cloud (as video recordings show very dramatically) and the specific effect on fire workers was to reduce lung function substantially, more than 12 times as much as would be expected in a group of similar age. The largest decline was among those who attended on the morning of September 11th. The exposure to dust was both massive and acute; while fire-fighters can be exposed to heavy smoke because of their regular work, and tend to recover from this, the overwhelming exposure on 9/11 has led to persistent reduction in lung function, with no prospect of recovery. Second, among almost 3300 office staff evacuated from the WTC virtually all (96%) reported at least one symptom of post-traumatic stress, with women, those on lower incomes, and those from ethnic minority groups at increased risk of post-traumatic stress disorder (Digrande et al. 2010). Understandably, those on higher floors, exposed to dust, and witnessing death or injury to others, were worst affected. Last, Claassen and her colleagues (2010) looked at the wider context; specifically, the impact of the attacks on rates of suicide in areas surrounding the three crash sites. There was no impact on suicide rates near the Pentagon or the Pennsylvania crash site, but rates within 150 miles of the WTC fell significantly in the six months after the attacks (and particularly two months after), compared with the previous six month period. The explanation, according to Claassen and her colleagues, lies in the increased social cohesion among those living in New York, a feature that Durkheim, over 100 years ago, pointed out led to a reduction in suicide rates.

All these health risks need to be set in context. DeHart (2003) observes that such risks pale in comparison with the very considerable benefits to travellers, and for business and international relations. But what of those who are not themselves travelling, but who may be impacted by those who are? What of more local impacts ('externality effects') on those who live close to airports, or under flight paths?

A good deal of research has been undertaken on the regional and local impacts of airports, specifically on exposure to noise and air pollution. This gains importance when there are plans to construct new airports or to expand existing facilities by building new runways. The noise and pollution arises not only from the aircraft themselves but also from the additional burden placed by road traffic in the vicinity of the airport. Stansfeld and his colleagues (Stansfeld et al. 2005, Clark et al. 2005) have examined the impact of exposure to aircraft (and associated road traffic) noise on the cognitive development of children attending schools near three European airports: London Heathrow; Amsterdam Schiphol; and Madrid Barajas. Over 2000 children aged 9-10 years, from 89 schools, formed the set of participants in the so-called RANCH study (Road traffic and Aircraft Noise exposure and children's Cognition and Health), and data comprised aircraft and road traffic noise exposure, together with survey data on health and cognitive outcomes (including reading comprehension, attention, and memory). Aircraft noise exposure (but not road traffic noise exposure) was associated with poor reading comprehension, even after allowance was made in the statistical analysis for socioeconomic variables (Figure 4.2). The fact that the results were consistent across all three international airports suggests that the findings are robust. While there did not appear to be significant impacts on overall mental health there is enough evidence for the authors to conclude that aircraft noise does impair cognitive development and that schools with high levels of exposure are not healthy educational environments.

This major study confirms the findings of earlier researchers. One longitudinal study (Hygge et al. 2002) into the cognitive performance of 326 children aged 9-13 years in Germany was made possible by a 'natural experiment', resulting from the closure of one airport in Munich and the opening of a new airport. Children in experimental groups had been exposed to noise from the new airport or were likely to be exposed to noise from the new airport. Two control groups were

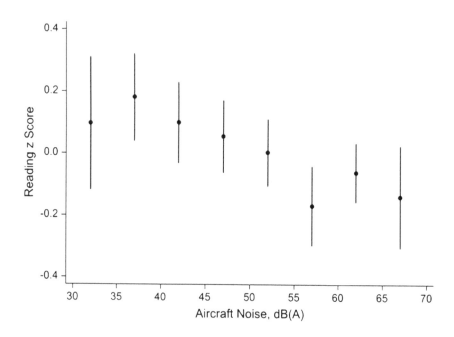

Figure 4.2   Mean reading scores (and confidence intervals) for children, by level of aircraft noise

Source: Reprinted with permission from Clark et al. (2005): 34.

selected from areas with little exposure to aircraft noise. Three waves of data were collected: six months prior to the changeover of airports, and one and two years later. Findings suggested that there was a significant deterioration in cognitive performance (long-term memory and reading ability) after the new airport had opened. At the old airport, children's cognitive performance improved after it had closed operations. The authors' work offers considerable support for the thesis that language processing is related to noise exposure, and that this could be reversed if noise was abated (Hygge et al. 2002: 473).

Other authors have looked at the health impacts among adult populations. Cohen et al. (2008) studied people living near La Guardia Airport in New York City and examined exposure both to noise and to particulate matter. Those living near the airport were exposed to four times the noise of those in quieter residential areas, and 55% of those living near the airport expressed annoyance with the noise, significantly more than those further away. Lin and colleagues (2008) have undertaken research on the association between proximity to airports and respiratory disease. Included in their study is La Guardia Airport, as well as two others in New York State. They found an increased risk of admission for respiratory conditions (asthma, chronic bronchitis) among residents living within

5 miles of the three airports (approximately 40% greater than compared with those living more than 5 miles away). However, it was not clear whether there was adequate control for confounding factors (such as housing quality or smoking in the home, since the domestic environment may have at least as much of an effect on respiratory health). Lars Jarup and his colleagues (2005, 2008) have studied the association between exposure to airport noise and hypertension (high blood pressure) and cardiovascular disease, in the vicinity of six European airports. They selected 6000 adults (aged 45-70 years) who had lived near airports for at least five years. They found significant relationships between the modelled exposure to both night-time air traffic noise and average daily road traffic noise, and risk of hypertension. This was after controlling for possible confounding factors. For aircraft noise, each 10-decibel increase led to a 14% increase in the risk of high blood pressure.

Finally, let me say something about recreational uses of the skies. In recent years parachuting (skydiving) has become a popular, if relatively expensive, recreational activity in the UK and elsewhere. Westman and Björnstig (2005) estimate that there are over 675,000 sports parachutists worldwide. Some choose to jump as a means of raising money for charity. Two studies in the UK have examined the cost to the NHS of injuries resulting from this activity. Lee and colleagues (1999) documented 174 jumpers who were injured at two Scottish parachute centres over five years, almost all of whom were first-time jumpers. Sixty-three per cent of those injured required hospital admission. The authors make the point that the amount raised for charity is very small in relation to the cost of treating those injured making their 'charity jumps', an argument supported by Baiju and James (2003). Westman and Björnstig (2005) cite evidence from the US that suggests over 500 people in the US died from injuries sustained in skydiving between 1986 and 2001. However, the authors themselves have undertaken an audit of Swedish data that suggests an improving safety record in that country. Specifically, the fatality rate dropped from 8.6 per 100,000 jumps in the 1960s to just 0.8 in the later 1990s (and this from a total of over 1.13 million jumps).

For completeness, reference should be made to accidents as a result of hot-air ballooning. These are relatively uncommon. For example, in the US between 1984 and 1988 there were 138 recorded crashes, and between 2000 and 2004 there were 86. The incidence was less common in the UK, with only 98 accidents over nearly 30 years; few of these accidents resulted in fatalities but those that did generally involved collisions with power lines (Hasham et al. 2004).

Concluding remarks

Travel by train, boat and air can all be enjoyed for its own sake. The mode of travel, and the journey itself, can – if the circumstances are right and particularly if one has the means to travel in some style – add to one's sense of well-being. But there are dis-benefits, either at the transport 'hub' (waiting for a delayed train, undergoing interminable safety checks at airports) or during the journey itself (such as unscheduled train stops, food-borne infections on ships, or new anxieties over air travel in a post 9/11 world). As with road travel, there are burdens of air pollution to acknowledge, and accidents on the journeys. But given the huge volumes of travel each year by these modes, the risks must be put into perspective. The journey, whether undertaken alone or as a communal activity, can be pleasurable and usually with a tangible outcome at the destination. With this in mind I now turn attention away from specific modes of travel to focus on a specific motivation for travel, namely tourism.

Chapter 5
Vacations and the Tourist

Introduction

Vacations can be taken relatively close to home, and tourist attractions can be enjoyed that are within only an hour or so of one's home. But my focus is primarily on vacations and tourist trips that involve overnight stay(s) and here I discuss the benefits conveyed by such trips, as well as the risks. A particular field of healthcare, travel medicine, has emerged in the last few years, with courses devoted to the subject, a professional study group (www.istm.org) and specialist journal (*Journal of Travel Medicine*) first published in 1994. As the name suggests, the focus of travel medicine is on developing guidelines for medical practitioners, and on promoting the development of safe and effective interventions. These are important scientific and policy areas, though my emphasis here is less on the biomedical and more on the social. I also concentrate on international rather than domestic patterns of tourism. The latter can, of course, be significant if one requires healthcare away from home and has to draw on health professionals with whom one is not registered.

Gushulak and MacPherson (2006) draw attention to the considerable growth in volume of international tourism in the last 60 years. Data from the World Tourism Organization suggest that the number of international tourist arrivals in 1950 was well under 50 million a year. By 2003 this had grown to almost 700 million, with Europe and the Americas the main destinations, although while their market share in 1950 was 95% this had dropped to 76% in 2000 as other destinations – notably South East Asia – had become more attractive.

What benefits and risks does travel to such destinations bring for the health and well-being of those on vacation? I examine first the extent to which vacation confers mental health benefits – perhaps simply by 'getting away from it all' or offering new environments to explore and enjoy. I also take the opportunity to explore the health consequences of a distinctive form of tourism – the pilgrimage. Next, I look at one specific risk encountered by some tourists, that due to over-exposure to the sun's radiation. In the final section I turn attention to those international tourists who seek sex rather than sun; aside from the obvious risks they may be subject to, I am particularly concerned with the wider health impacts on local populations who may be exploited by such tourists.

Vacations and mental health

Vacations were, for many years, the prerogative of the well-to-do who could afford the time and cost to travel to spas and springs for rest and recuperation. By the start of the 20th century vacationing was a means for the middle classes to improve their physical health and add to their emotional well-being (Gini 2003: 52). It was not until the 1930s, in the US and UK, that vacationing became a way of life for the wider workforce. In the US, travel by automobile has always been the mode of choice, with 80% of vacationing Americans taking the car on their trip. Gini (2003) traces, albeit in a very anecdotal way, the changing nature of the vacation experience in the post-war US. Automobile travel on vacation, before the extensive network of interstate highways was constructed, was somewhat basic, with poor quality 'motor courts' or cabins for stop-overs and 'a Texaco gas station with dirty bathrooms and a Coca-Cola machine which was invariably empty or broken' (Gini 2003: 44). Motel chains that emerged later were, he suggests, clean and reasonably priced, even if homogeneous in appearance.

In order to assess the benefits of vacations for physical health Gump and Matthews (2000) examine the multiple risk factors associated with coronary heart disease among middle-aged men in the US. Participants were asked if they had had one or more vacations during the previous 12 months and the men were followed up over 5 years, during which some died. Those who had had at least one vacation were significantly less likely to have died from cardiovascular disease during the study period, even after allowing for possible confounding factors. Research from scientists working at the Alpine Medicine and Tourism Health Unit in Innsbruck, Austria, confirms that active vacations at moderate altitudes (up to 1700m) offer significant improvements in obesity and hypertension among overweight men (Strauss-Blasche et al. 2004, Schobersberger et al. 2009).

Strauss-Blasche and colleagues (2005) looked at what kinds of vacation characteristics predict good health outcomes following the vacation. They studied just under 200 white-collar workers, finding that health was improved if one had sufficient free time to oneself, enough time to exercise, opportunity to make new acquaintances, and a warmer and sunnier vacation setting. Health outcomes were worse the great the time-difference from home and if the weather during the vacation was poor. These findings are unsurprising. Many of us have had negative experiences journeying to and from the vacation destination, as well as during it; lost or delayed luggage, lost passports, poor-quality hotels, family arguments, and so on all create more stress than may have arisen in the absence of the vacation! In an earlier study (Strauss-Blasche et al. 2000), the same authors looked at how long the positive effects of a vacation lasted, for a cohort of Austrian employees. They recorded the number of physical complaints, the quality of sleep, and mood, 10 days before, and 3 days and 5 weeks after a vacation, noting that even five weeks after returning respondents reported fewer physical complaints than before the holiday.

In a recent meta-analysis of studies of vacation effects on health and well-being, de Bloom and colleagues (2009) are critical of many such studies, arguing that more robust designs are needed to assess such effects, with good data taken before, during, and after, the vacation. It is not always clear whether improvements in health and well-being are due to the vacation itself or to some other cause. Such studies as exist do, they argue nonetheless, suggest that vacations confer moderate positive benefits on both physical health and mental well-being ('re-charging one's batteries'), but that such effects are of short duration (lasting typically 2-4 weeks) once work is resumed.

The blurring of boundaries between working hours and non-working hours – made possible by new communications technologies – has, for some people, become a feature of contemporary life (Lyons and Urry 2005). With the increasing ubiquity of email and mobile phones it is easy to 'connect' outside the workplace and to continue work-related conversations into the evenings and weekends. This extends to vacations; plenty of us will have had the experience of being asked if we are contactable while on vacation ('will you be answering emails?'). Gini (2003: 58) suggests that 40% of Americans are at work when not in the office, remaining in daily contact via email and mobile phone from their vacation cabins. He cites a Chief Executive: 'You just keep doing what you do, just from a different location. With e-mail, faxes and cell phones, you'd have to go to the South Pacific Islands to truly get away from your job' (Gini 2008: 62). Surely, for the sake of proper rest and recuperation, there is a time (and a place) to 'switch off' in order to reduce stress, renew relationships and return to work refreshed? There are times, surely, when being dis-connected and sedentary is an attractive proposition.

Some opportunities to 'switch off' might usefully be taken on one's own. For some people, solitary travelling and vacationing can be genuinely therapeutic, providing the opportunity to collect thoughts and to reflect on problems and issues, perhaps on a long walk. While there is plenty of evidence that social contact and social networks are health-promoting, in certain circumstances solitude can offer inner peace and self-discovery. As Thoreau (cited in Long et al. 2003) observed, 'I never found the companion that was so companionable as solitude'. These positive aspects of solitude can be realised in many different environments. For the students surveyed by Long and his colleagues (2003) their home (dormitory/apartment) was the most common setting for solitude, but natural environments were also conducive to feelings of anonymity, creativity and self-discovery. Indeed, the Wilderness Act of 1964 in the US was introduced in part to preserve natural environments but also to provide opportunities for solitude. As Long et al. (2003: 580) observe: 'Psychology's almost exclusive emphasis on *loneliness*... seems disproportionate' (my emphasis). One can be alone without feeling lonely.

Recent years have seen the rise of the active vacation, whether this means working on a kibbutz, an archaeological dig, or taking part in extreme sports, some of which demand time and money (and good health!). In some instances the activity is established *explicitly* to provide therapy. There is a considerable literature on the therapeutic benefits of getting people (usually troubled adolescents) to experience, and be active in, natural environments such as national parks or wilderness areas (Ewert et al. 2003). Terms used include 'wilderness therapy' or 'adventure therapy'. Such organised excursions and programmes have become well-established in North America and parts of Europe. For example, the adventure programme 'Outward Bound', established by the German educator Kurt Hahn in the 1940s, was based on challenging expeditions in wilderness areas (Ewert et al. 2003). Building on this, many programmes in the US and other countries of the global north employ a medical model that involves clinicians and therapists to help people with behavioural problems or learning disabilities. Ewert and his colleagues suggest that some ten thousand adolescents each year are involved in wilderness therapy in the US. They report on climbing expeditions in the French Alps for adults with learning disabilities and wilderness programmes on remote islands off New Zealand for Maori adolescents.

Such programmes may lead to great self-control ('self-efficacy') and reduced incidence of depression and anxiety, but there does not seem to be, as yet, a secure evidence base for this kind of intervention. It is not clear whether any benefits to health and well-being derive from (some or all of) being transported and connected to a very different environment, engaging in unfamiliar physical activity, or being part of a larger (and also unfamiliar) social group with set 'boundaries' on behaviour. At times, the popular press castigates health agencies and social workers for 'wasting' public money on 'fun' activities for those who should not – they would argue – be rewarded with such 'treats'.

It does seem reasonable to suggest that contact with nature, whether in urban parks, forests, or wilderness areas, is important for one's sense of well-being, helping to reduce stress in working lives and improve mental health. Nature 'restores'; but simply being away may be enough to detach oneself from the stresses of contemporary living. In other contexts the same holds true; for example, in a study of people with physical impairments who experience respite care, Conradson (2005) finds gains in physical energy and emotional benefit from leaving behind the pace of daily life and being able to enjoy green space, relative peace and perhaps the chance to come into contact with animals.

There is a tension between maintaining wilderness areas and providing access to such areas for public benefit (Peters 2006: Chapter 4). For example, the National Park Service in the US undertook 'Mission 66', designed to provide better car access to major national parks (such as Yosemite and Yellowstone). This opened up such parks to many more people who will have benefited from their experiences of perhaps previously unknown attractions. Others, however, want the 'authentic' wilderness experience and, for them, the opening up of access and the short visit simply to 'tick' a place as visited, is anathema. The physical effort or energy expended in reaching the destination (driving, taking a train, bus or plane) is modest in relation to that in the wilderness destination itself (such as walking, hiking, or canoeing, all of which involve body-work). As Waskul and Waskul (2009) observe in relation to their shared journeys by canoe in the Minnesota wilderness, in addition to canoeing and carrying the canoe, effort is needed to subsist (fish, collect wood, build a fire); work ('travail') is required. And there are benefits to accompany this work: 'well into the evening around the campfire, we discuss at length our affective and emotional experiences as we anticipate our return to normative everyday life' (Waskul and Waskul 2009: 35). Further benefits for this couple are the strengthening of their relationship and the freedom from everyday concerns: 'We can't do it alone. We have to rely on one another. And I love that there is no cell phone, no computer, no TV'(Waskul and Waskul 2009: 35).

Much of what is discussed in this chapter relates to the individual, or family, or perhaps small group travelling abroad. But there is one class of mobility that is of a very different purpose and scale, and this is the pilgrimage. Having examined whether vacations are good for mental health, what are the health benefits (and risks) of going on pilgrimage? Pilgrimage involves the individual religious devotee, or perhaps small group, travelling to a holy place or shrine that is believed to be sacred. For example, people have for years travelled to Lourdes to pray for better health or a cure for disease (see Gesler 1996, for an examination of Lourdes and other holy sites as therapeutic landscapes).

For the pilgrim, travelling to a sacred place delivers a spiritual benefit – a mental health gain, one might say – from both the journey and the destination, even if serious physical effort might be involved. 'Contrary to the ideal of effortless transportation, a pilgrimage is normally connected with certain physical difficulties that the pilgrim has to endure' (Melin 2008: 93). This contrasts with the package holiday; a 'quick win' as it were. For the 'eco-theological' Christian pilgrim the journey on foot represents a means of 'reconquering slowness' (Melin 2008: 95). Indeed, Melin goes so far (!) as to suggest that pilgrimage could usefully be seen as a metaphor to encourage people to adapt their travel behaviours away from polluting modes of transport towards more carbon-free modes.

As Gushulak and MacPherson (2006: 307) note, pilgrimages often involve very large group gatherings. For example, Kumbh Mela is a pilgrimage that sees millions of Hindus gather to bathe in the River Ganges; over 10 million pilgrims visited in 2001, including 1 million people from outside India. Inevitably, such a massive gathering has health implications. At the 1954 Kumbh Mela in Allahabad, around 500 people were killed, and many more injured in a stampede. Gushulak and MacPherson refer to accidental death by drowning as a common occurrence but there does not seem to be data on how common this is.

Better known, perhaps, are the Hajj pilgrimages to Mecca, involving many more international visitors. Two million people visit the Muslim holy city on five specified days each year, some spending up to a month engaged in prayer and ritual (Ahmed et al. 2006). Over the course of the Hajj, a pilgrim may travel over 80 km across different sites to retrace the footsteps of the Prophet Mohammed, with most pilgrims covering some part of this distance on foot. Clingingsmith et al. (2008) suggest that the Hajj may help forge a common Islamic identity, with no evidence that this is defined in opposition to non-Muslims; the notions of equality and harmony tend to extend to members of other religions. Ahmed and colleagues (2006) have focused more on the health risks, suggesting that the extreme congestion of accommodation and Hajj activities increase the risks of injury and infectious disease. Pilgrims arriving from areas of high endemicity for tuberculosis (see Chapter 9) have led to the prevalence of TB being three times as great in Mecca compared with elsewhere in Saudi Arabia. Respiratory tract infections are common during the Hajj, with estimates of up to 24,000 possible cases of influenza in 2003. As with Kumbh Mela there is the risk of stampede; one in 2006 killed 380 and wounded 289 pilgrims, while 251 died in a stampede in 2004. As Ahmed and colleagues observe, managing the Hajj and its vast mobile population is a monumental task for the Saudi authorities.

Those who have travelled to resource-poor countries will be familiar with travellers' diarrhoea (TD), which can emerge after 3-4 days' stay and last for about four days if untreated. TD is usually transmitted as a result of the faecal contamination of foodstuffs and drinks; the most common pathogen is *Escherichia coli* (*E coli*) but infection by *Salmonella* or *Shigella* is also found. The risks vary geographically. Those visiting western and northern Europe, or North America, or Australasia have incidence rates of less than 8%, while rates of TD between 8-20% are observed in southern Europe, South Africa and Japan. In the developing world the rates can be up to 60% during the first two weeks' stay (Steffen et al. 2003).

Studies of the risks of returning home with various illnesses have been undertaken over many years. A European network of clinicians interested in travel medicine has created 'EuroTravNet' (www.eurotravenet.eu) and data for 2008 on almost 7000 European travellers have been analysed by Field and her colleagues (2010). These indicate that gastrointestinal disease accounts for one-third of all illnesses, though concern is expressed about imported cases of malaria (see Chapter 9). A survey of those returning via Cardiff Airport in Wales in 2001 found that about one-quarter of almost 1500 people reported diarrhoea and a similar proportion reported sunburn; about 8% reported respiratory infections (Evans et al. 2001). Rates of illness were higher among those who had made late bookings and varied with destination; thus the odds of diarrhoea were significantly higher when returning from the Canary Islands, Cyprus and Bulgaria. Some of these illnesses can be self-managed but Evans et al. (2001) suggests that one in five overseas travellers consults a general practitioner (GP) on returning home, and this is a considerable burden on the health service if we consider the number of holiday trips taken abroad each year.

In a more broadly-based study of a range of infectious gastrointestinal diseases (IGD) Swaminathan and colleagues (2009) drew on data from a network of surveillance centres that reported on problems that were sufficiently serious to merit a clinical consultation on return home. Not all the travellers were tourists (though two-thirds were). Results suggested that over a quarter (29%) of returned travellers had a diagnosis of IGD; of these, younger travellers, those who were tourists, and women were most at risk. Infection with *Campylobacter* and *Giardia* were most prevalent, and the most common 'source' regions were South Asia, South America, and the Middle East.

Table 5.1   **Age-adjusted incidence of malignant melanoma (per 100,000 persons), 1975-2005**

Country		1975	1985	1995	2005
Australia	Males	n.d	33.9	52.1	61.5
	Females	n.d.	31.2	37.0	42.8
USA	Males	9.2	13.7	20.7	25.8
	Females	7.4	10.9	13.7	17.2
Britain	Males	2.5	4.8	7.9	13.4
	Females	3.9	7.8	10.3	14.6

Sources: Australian Institute for Health & Welfare; SEER Cancer Statistics (US); Cancer Research UK.

Note: n.d. means no data available.

Sun exposure

It is well-known that exposure to the sun increases the risk of skin cancer. But such exposure can be frequent (chronic) or infrequent (intermittent) and there are different types of skin cancer. Of the latter, melanoma is the most serious, and it accounts for about 80% of deaths from skin cancer.

Data on the incidence of malignant melanoma reveal geographical and gender differences, as well as increasing incidence over the last 35 years (Table 5.1). Australia has the highest rates in the world, and has seen the incidence rise since the 1980s. In the US incidence has also increased sharply and, as in Australia, is higher among men than women. Incidence in Britain has also risen since 1975 but has always been higher among women than men.

To what extent can the incidence, and the increasing incidence, of malignant melanoma, be attributed to sun exposure as a result of travel? There is a good deal of evidence to suggest that intermittent exposure causes melanoma, and that such exposure arises during recreational activities and vacations. This intermittent exposure, it is argued, causes genomic damage (to DNA), particularly during childhood and adolescence (Oliviera et al. 2006), though not all epidemiologists agree about this. One study offering support for the hypothesis conducted a case-control analysis (cases of malignant melanoma, controls were healthy adults) in Ontario, Canada (Walter et al. 1999). This suggested (Table 5.2) that having had beach vacations at ages 12 and 18 were significant risk factors for the disease, unlike more recent beach vacations or chronic exposure (regular outdoor exposure, where the exposure seems protective of skin cancer). The significance of these ages lies in the fact that adolescents and young adults are at risk because of intense sun exposure, particularly in tropical areas (O'Riordan et al. 2008). Although a generalisation, their intention is to return home with a suntan, and the risk of sunburn is one that some are prepared to take. O'Riordan and his colleagues estimate that a three-week vacation in Hawaii can potentially double the annual dose of ultraviolet radiation.

Further support for the intermittent exposure hypothesis comes from research undertaken on young German children (aged 6 or 7 years). This suggests (Gefeller et al. 2007) that those children who have spent more family vacations in sunny, Mediterranean areas show a statistically significant increase in the numbers of melanocytic 'nevi'; conversely, those children whose vacations have been on the North Sea or Baltic Sea show no association between increasing frequency of vacations and numbers of nevi. Such nevi are thought to be the precursors to melanoma and possibly a first step in the development of malignant melanoma.

Table 5.2   Relative risk of melanoma associated with intermittent exposure

Type of exposure	Odds ratio (95% confidence interval)
Beach vacation in past 5 years	1.04 (0.82-1.32)
Beach vacations at age 12 years	1.67 (1.31-2.12)
Beach vacations at age 18 years	1.29 (1.00-1.67)
Outdoor activity between ages 10 and 20 years (>100 days a year)	0.67 (0.52-0.85)

Source: Walter et al. (1999: 420)

Although indirect evidence of an association, rather than a causal explanation, Agredano and colleagues (2006) have suggested that increasing passenger travel by air corresponds closely to the increasing incidence noted in Table 5.1. Cheaper winter travel to warmer destinations has, they argue, increased exposure to UV radiation.

Sex tourism

While travel overseas primarily for the purpose of seeking sexual services is nothing new, the availability of cheap air travel has rendered quite accessible a range of destinations, mostly though not exclusively in the global south, as sites for such consumption. Any deep understanding of sex tourism draws upon several of the 'mobilising concepts' introduced in Chapter 1, particularly networks, globalisation and inequality. I focus initially on the *purchase* of sexual services though, clearly, there is much to be said about the health impacts of tourism in which sex is part of a broader pattern of consuming a lifestyle based on sun, sand and sea.

As Hesse and his colleagues (2008) observe, very large numbers of young people go abroad on vacation each year, attracted particularly to resorts that have a reputation for partying. Several studies have shown that consumption of alcohol and drugs increases during such vacations, though this varies according to setting. According to Hesse and colleagues young British travellers to Ibiza have a high consumption of drugs while young British backpackers in Australia are more likely to consume alcohol. Hesse's own study is of young Danish people travelling to a Black Sea resort, on trips organised by agencies specialising in 'party packages' where the representatives' role is actively to encourage hedonism. As one rep puts it: 'We tell them at our meeting to just let go. They should do whatever they want. It's their free choice because they've paid for their vacation. Down here there are no rules. So they should take advantage of that' (Hesse et al. 2008). And take advantage they clearly do. The young people they surveyed seem to drink 12 or more units of alcohol each day during their vacation (the recommended daily amounts are 3-4 units for men and 2-3 units for women). The suggested strategies, back home, after a night out partying (take a taxi, contact the police) are not always the safest ones abroad, where taxi drivers may demand high prices, may harass the passengers and try to sell illegal drugs, and (in the Bulgarian resort Hesse's team studied) the police are – they assert – not an authority to be trusted.

Wonders and Michalowski (2001) couch sex tourism firmly within a structuralist framework. They argue that the forces of globalisation 'shape the consumption of sexual services by fostering tourism as an industry aimed at those who have the resources to travel and purchase what they desire, thus facilitating the commodification of both male desire and women's bodies within the global capitalist economy' (Wonders and Michalowski 2001: 546). They acknowledge that there are wealthy North American and European women seeking sex from young men in resource-poor countries, men wanting to purchase services, and women selling their bodies. Sex tourism is seen as one aspect of the global movements of bodies, whether for business or pleasure, not simply a problem caused by prostitutes. As they put it, 'privileged bodies from industrialized nations cross into less developed ones in search of exotic pleasures and a little (highly controlled) danger' (Wonders and Michalowski 2001: 548). Other bodies are enjoyed (consumed) by those who regard them as material manifestations of an exotic cultural fantasy, one that can never be realised at home. Men (often white) can exercise their supremacy over females (usually non-white), perhaps in former colonial settings. Sex tourism is therefore both racialised and gendered consumption, and (as the authors put it neatly) women themselves become the tourist destination.

This broad canvas is revealed sharply in both Amsterdam and Havana. Thirty years ago there was substantial immigration to the Netherlands from former Dutch colonies such as Surinam, followed more recently by people from Africa, South America and the former Soviet Union, all seeking economic improvement. Virtually half the population of Amsterdam comprises migrants. Unemployment among these residents is high and economic prospects poor, helping to drive women into prostitution. The sex industry is organised and controlled (as well as regulated by legislation), and oriented towards meeting the desires of, in the main, foreign leisure and business travellers. In Havana prostitution re-emerged in the 1990s after years of US embargos that restricted tourism to Cuba. Growth in the tourist industry was also a response to the economic decline in state-sector employment associated with a post-socialist world. The legalisation of the American dollar allowed the growing number of sex workers to secure hard currency from tourists for their services, without breaking the law. In addition, Wonders and Michalowski suggest that Havana prostitutes operated more independently and the 'reasonable' rates they charged permitted men to spend more time in their company, providing an experience that was less like a quick commercial transaction. While the forces of globalisation are creating new sites for sex work, local conditions shape how that work is produced and consumed.

Wonders and Michalowski do not concern themselves directly with issues of risk, health and well-being, other than noting in conclusion that further increases in tourist sex will be at the expense of the welfare and health of those meeting the demands of wealthy foreigners. We need, therefore, to ask what risks to health and well-being emerge as a result of these transactions? In western countries, notably the Netherlands, sex tourism is tightly controlled by the government; this means that HIV rates are low among workers in the industry. But in the global south regulation is less common and such workers find themselves marginalised and disempowered. Here, women may benefit slightly from the financial transactions (though much will be extracted by the men who control them) but in making, at best, enough to get by, they often put themselves at risk of physical abuse and mental stress.

Several of the essays in the collection edited by Thomas and her colleagues (2010) address these themes. Consider three of the studies. Padilla and Castellanos (2010) examine the 'touristic borderlands' of the Dominican Republic, where 'impoverished service workers who are functionally excluded from global mobility intermingle with a wide range of global "elites", for whom such mobility is a taken-for-granted source of pride and modern social capital' (Padilla and Castellanos 2010: 91). Their ethnographic work reveals patterns of internal migration, by young men who become sex workers, to places designated as tourist 'growth poles'. The lucrative exchanges of money for sex offer what is for most the unrealistic prospect of leaving the country in the company of wealthy women who have sought their services. The men assess the risk of HIV infection according to context; sex with women tourists at the beach was designated as riskier (and hence resulted in use of condoms) than in their local neighbourhoods. In a related paper Padilla, Guilamo-Ramos and their colleagues (2010) suggest that between 50,000 and 250,000 women are sex workers in the Dominican Republic, and that such work overlaps, as it does for male sex workers, with other employment. Migration is both internal and overseas, as men and women develop relationships with clients that involve emotional and financial exchanges (leading to 'trust' and therefore lack of protection) that generate trips abroad. As the authors express it: 'The transnational connections between the Dominican Republic and other countries therefore constitute a highly permeable air bridge through which both people and microbes can move' (Padilla et al. 2010: 73). Domestically, as noted in other contexts, migrants arriving in the capital (Santo Domingo) may engage in risky sexual behaviours before returning to infect partners in rural hinterlands.

In a similar study – also countering the usual focus on male tourists exploiting local women – Nyanzi and Bah (2010) focus on male 'bumsters' in the Gambia and their relations with female tourists (the vast majority from western Europe). Contrary to popular imaginings, these men are not always destitute and uneducated; yet their use of condoms depended upon the tourist partners' preferences. Nyanzi and Bah query the inequalities: 'if the fantasised sexual services of a black man are received in exchange for the dream of a plane ticket to an imagined West, who is exploiting who?' (Nyanzi and Bah, 2010: 118). In a third study, Schifter and Thomas (2010) look at the sex industry in Costa Rica. As in the Dominican Republic the pattern is one of internal migration of young men and women to the capital, San José, where they engage in sex work. As in the Gambia, they are not always uneducated and impoverished, but unlike the Gambia the sex work is mostly directed at wealthy American men who find the 'exotic look' rather different from that they might encounter back home.

Clearly, sex workers in countries such as these have some 'agency'; they are not necessarily coerced into prostitution, which may be, for them, a legitimate means of earning a living (Gatrell 2010). A sex worker who has some control over her working conditions may be more likely to access health care as the need arises. A converse view, which would certainly be more appropriate in understanding 'trafficking', is that such women are exploited and, controlled by male pimps, wholly disempowered. I return to this theme in the next chapter.

While *child* sex tourism is a relatively under-research area (Lau 2008) many of the determinants are similar to those involving exploited adults. Children as well as adults are trafficked across international borders, while the exoticism of the 'other' (especially the oriental other) applies to children too. Thailand has, for some years, had a reputation as a destination for the sex tourist interested in accessing vulnerable children, such access being facilitated by organised gangs, corrupt local politicians, legal officials and even parents (Lau 2008). It is, Lau argues, relatively easy (aided by new web and communications technologies) to secure the sexual services of children, with the government not doing enough to prevent such exploitation, since tourism revenue is an important part of the economy. The UK campaign group End Child Prostitution, Child Pornography and the Trafficking of Children for Sexual Purposes, ECPAT (www.ecpat.org. uk/sites/default/files/thailand05.pdfECPAT) suggests it accounts for some 6% of Thailand's GDP. Some exploiters are opportunistic but others are paedophiles very familiar with beach resorts (such as Pattaya and Phuket) and the capital, Bangkok. ECPAT suggests that, to avoid detection, children are rotated around the country's tourist destinations.

This exploitation leads to physical and emotional problems for the children involved, putting them at risk of infection, violence, substance abuse, mental illness, and unwanted pregnancies (and therefore the risks of 'backstreet' abortions). Young prostitutes who have been infected are often returned home having had no medical treatment, and this mobility can expose other populations to risk. Again, in structuralist terms this particular form of sex tourism, fuelled by the purchasing power of foreign tourists, perpetuates inequality and disparities of power (Lau 2008).

Concluding remarks

Millions of people go on vacation each year, whether in family groups, small parties, or as lone travellers. Their experiences can be socially and culturally rich and they can return refreshed. This is likely to be the common pattern, and the ordinariness of the vacation means that academic attention focuses less on the positive health aspects of tourism and more on the risks to health. These risks can include accidents, infections, and – depending on the destination – over-exposure to the sun. But it bears repeating that, in general, tourism induces health and well-being for the individual.

As we have seen, however, the traveller is not the only one exposed to risk. Those who are taken advantage of by the tourist, especially in unequal sexual relationships, may themselves be subject to considerable risk. I turn in the next chapter to mobilities and health risks among the dispossessed, those most othered of others who may be subject to extreme risks.

Part 2: Migration

Migration can take place over a variety of geographic scales, including short-distance relocation, within-country moves from one region to another, and from one country to another. In the case of international migration there may well be pressure to adapt to a new cultural environment in order to feel accepted by the host population; most obviously, this will express itself where there is a need to learn a new language. Social scientists have, for many years, sought to understand processes of assimilation or acculturation and I touch on these issues here where there are obvious health dimensions. Note also that there are different definitions of a 'migrant' in an international context. Sometimes this refers solely to people born overseas (first-generation migrants) but some studies also include persons with one or both parents born overseas (second-generation migrants).

The volume and scale of voluntary migration should not be under-estimated. For example, within the US about 23% of the population aged over 65 years of age moved between 1995 and 2000; this is close to 2 million persons. But these figures are dwarfed within China, where (according to the 2000 Census) there were over 120 million internal migrants, mostly moving from rural to urban areas (Wen et al. 2010: 453).

There is a rich tradition of research on the relationship between migration and health, with several overviews (see, for example, Gushalak and MacPherson 2006). Much of this literature is medical in focus, examining the impacts that immigrants have on health services and the infections they may transmit when they arrive at new destinations. Other work looks at the extent to which migration offers a 'natural experiment' in assessing the relative importance of genetics and environment in disease causation.

I shall consider some of this research in the next two chapters but I also want to consider the inequalities that arise. In particular, and in contrast with much of the 'mobilities' literature, I examine the experiences and health status of those whose mobility is not of their choosing but where circumstances of conflict or poverty force them from their homes or require them to seek improvements in their lives by moving elsewhere. Here, the forces of globalisation impact directly on millions of people, many trafficked across borders and exploited ruthlessly by gangs who use modern technologies to organise their activities. Others are forced to move, some permanently, some temporarily, by disasters or by major development projects from which they derive little or no benefit, only cost.

Cresswell (2006: 25) suggests that 'in contemporary social thought, words associated with mobility are unremittingly positive. If something can be said to be fluid, dynamic, in flux, or simply mobile, then it is seen to be progressive, exciting, and contemporary'. He contrasts this with those things that are fixed, static, bounded or rooted – and consequently 'dull'. But he also makes the point that our understanding of mobility has changed over time. Certainly in the contemporary UK and France there is a sense in which migration is 'bad' for the economy and society; (in)migration has almost become a dirty word. In the UK groups such as MigrationWatch put inward migration firmly at the top of the political agenda, while the forced removal of 'undesirable' Roma people from France hit the headlines in summer 2010. At all costs, it seems, governments are bent on keeping the wrong people from crossing borders and contaminating the domestic sphere. The popular press continues to use aquatic metaphors (swamp, flood, tidal wave, surge) or biological ones (swarm, flock, blight) to demonise those who may bring infections with them (Ingram 2008: 882).

Chapter 6
The Displaced and the Dispossessed

Introduction

As shown in previous chapters there are undoubtedly risks incurred in journeying from place to place. Yet these journeys and encounters pale into insignificance compared with what I want to deal with here, which is to focus on the health of the forcibly displaced. Such groups include: those who are displaced by war and conflict, either within or across national borders; those displaced by development projects; those displaced by natural disasters; and those who are 'trafficked' from one country to another. Here, there is little human agency or choice; the 'push' factors trump the 'pull' factors (Kemp and Rasbridge 2004). The burden of such displacements falls very much on the most marginal, disadvantaged and vulnerable populations since the better-off will, in many circumstances (but not all) have the resources to deal with the consequences.

The importance of the task is captured vividly in this quotation from the Palestinian writer Edward Said, taken from Cresswell (2002: 16):

> For surely it is one of the unhappiest characteristics of the age to have produced more refugees, migrants, displaced persons, and exiles than ever before in history, most of them as an accompaniment to and, ironically enough, as afterthoughts of great post-colonial and imperial conflicts. As the struggle for independence produced new states and new boundaries, it also produced homeless wanderers, nomads, vagrants, unassimilated to the emerging structures of institutional power, rejected by the established order for their intransigence and obdurate rebelliousness.

Displaced persons are not a modern phenomenon. So I start this chapter with a brief examination of the African slave trade and its impacts on indigenous populations before looking at the health impacts of those trafficked in more contemporary settings.

From slavery to human trafficking

If we seek an historical perspective on the associations between forced movement and ill-health the trans-Atlantic slave trade between the 15th and 19th centuries provides graphic material. This trade was motivated by the need for labour to work on plantations (such as cotton and coffee), in mines, and in domestic service, in the Americas. Historians (for example, Klein 1999, and Thomas 1997) continue to debate the levels of mortality during the Atlantic crossings. Mortality rates appear to have depended on the length of the voyage, the port of origin, the carrier country, the demographic composition of the slaves, ship size and, crucially, the health status of the slaves before they embarked. For example, some ports in Africa were more affected than others by yellow fever and malaria, while local food crises weakened slaves before they were transported. Klein (1999: 130-8) suggests that while mortality rates on the voyage could be extremely high (over 50% on some ships) in general mortality rates were of the order of 15% in the 17th century and 3% in the 19th century. But he also suggests that mortality was much higher among slaves being transported overland to the African coast for shipment overseas.

Among those who had to endure the Atlantic crossing the main cause of ill-health (and mortality) was dysentery, while deaths were also due in no small measure to smallpox. Smallpox had been introduced into the Americas in the early 16th century by the Spanish conquest of Mexico, and in the 16th, 17th and 18th centuries by the slave trade that brought west Africans to Spanish Hispaniola (modern Haiti and the Dominican Republic) and to the Portuguese colony of Brazil. The smallpox virus is transmitted by droplets exhaled by infectives and inhaled by susceptibles, and was unknown in the Americas before Europeans arrived. Alden and Miller (1987) examine how the slave trade helped to transmit smallpox to Brazil over a 250 year period (1560 through to 1831). Drought and crop failures brought refugees to west African cities, and many of these refugees (tens of thousand each year) found themselves transported involuntarily to Brazil to work in the cane sugar plantations. When they reached one of the Brazilian ports, if infected they spread contagion rapidly from the waterside sheds in which they waited to be auctioned off. From the seaports the disease diffused rapidly along trails and inland waterways.

Klein concludes his discussion of slave mortality by observing that infectious disease was not the only cause; on-board rebellions and suicides also contributed. He further notes that the vast majority of slaves did indeed reach the Americas. Somewhat surprisingly, he suggests that, 'despite this atmosphere of violence, the experience may not have been as psychologically damaging as some have claimed' (Klein 1999: 159). Slave traders wanted to maximise profits and it was in their interest to deliver a healthy new workforce. But we need to contrast this perspective with the horrific descriptions (Thomas 1997: 422-8) of how slave rebellions were quashed, and the protagonists dealt with. Simply observing that most slaves survived does little to counter the obvious point that these vast numbers of people were stripped of their dignity, well-being, and rights to live a free life. They were surely the 'other' *par excellence*. Ironically, it was the high death rates among crew that were used by some abolitionists to argue for the ending of the slave trade.

I considered in Chapter 5 the issue of sex work as it related to mobility, noting that while there was evidence of exploitation there was in some cases the exercising of choice or agency. In the case of human trafficking it is difficult to imagine the operation of any agency at all (Gatrell 2010). The UN defines human trafficking as: 'the recruitment, transportation, transfer, harbouring or receipt of persons by means of threat or use of force' (Miller et al. 2007: 486). It is exceptionally difficult to collect reasonably accurate data on the numbers of people trafficked across international borders, or, indeed, within countries, but the UN suggests that the figure is up to a million persons a year. The 'traffic' generates some £12 billion income each year (Gatrell 2010: 220). While Hodge (2008: 144) cites a figure of up to 17,500 persons, Miller and her colleagues suggest that some 50,000 women and children are trafficked annually into the US, treated as commercial objects and subject to enormous risks. Women and children from a wide range of ethnic backgrounds are trafficked, with sexually exploited children from 40 different countries identified in one study (Hodge 2008).

Regardless of the figure, the problem is serious. Some women may travel voluntarily, in that they are promised employment as domestic servants, waitresses or in factories, but on arrival can find themselves in debt bondage, required to pay extortionate sums to those who have brought them in. If they default they are coerced into sex work, required to engage in sex with strangers many times a day. Tracing them becomes difficult if they are moved 'to keep fresh faces at sex work venues and also to inhibit women's ability to gain social support ... and to reduce their access to assistance' (Miller et al. 2007: 488). The health consequences are many. For example, there are physical and psychological impacts due to the violence that may be encountered during the trafficking. Substance abuse goes hand-in-hand with the introduction to sex work. Serious mental health problems arise from exposure to violence and threats.

Evidence suggests that it is the most vulnerable that get trafficked; the poor, or orphaned, or illiterate, taken from resource-poor countries. Consider, for example, India, where Joffres and her colleagues (2008) estimate that up to 20,000 Bangladeshi women and girls, and up to 10,000 Nepalis are trafficked into India each year, many of the latter from ethnic minority groups living in remote hill villages or impoverished border communities. As Hodge (2008: 144) puts it, 'a girl might be kidnapped from a village in Nepal, trafficked to India and sold for $1,000 and then trafficked to the United States and sold for $20,000 or more'. In such resource-poor countries the economic and political circumstances are such that environments are created in which it becomes possible and profitable for traffickers to recruit children and women. But the trafficking is not always across international borders. Joffres et al. (2008) suggest that 89% of the trafficking of children and women in India for commercial sexual exploitation is between states, with rural states meeting the 'needs' in Delhi, Kolkata and Mumbai. Those trafficked find themselves working not only in traditional city brothels but also in bars and clubs along the main national highways.

The appalling burdens of such trafficking are brought into sharp relief with a case study reported by Miller and her colleagues (2007). This relates to a 27 year old Guatemalan woman who had paid $10,000 to a group of *coyotes* (those facilitating illegal migration) to engineer a move to Boston and whose struggles to pay back the money resulted in threats of violence to family members back home and led to involvement in a prostitute ring. Thus, although not trafficked for sex *per se*, there is evidence of profound vulnerability, set within the context of impoverishment. Lack of personal documentation resulted in her invisibility as far as the US health-care system was concerned, her case only coming to light when her sister-in-law brought her to an antenatal clinic. Stories such as this bring home the true nature of the violence – symbolic and real – done to many women from the global south.

In the case of children, the number being trafficked is difficult to measure with any accuracy. Beyrer (2004) suggests that between 1 and 1.2 million children a year are trafficked globally, with a focus on West Africa, eastern Europe (trafficking into western Europe), Mexico and Colombia (into the US). Most are trafficked for cheap labour but others for adoption, arranged marriages, sexual exploitation or the 'harvesting' of organs. Of these, Beyrer highlights the demand for child labour, noting that the trafficked numbers are a tiny proportion of the estimated 246 million child labourers across the globe. In Africa, many children are coerced into joining paramilitary organisations and forced into landmine clearance and sexual activity.

As Biemann (2002) and others have noted, sex tourism and the worldwide trafficking of women have been assisted by some of the correlates of globalization, including the rise of the information society and the changing economic relations in south-east Asia; these processes have contributed to the ease with which female bodies can be trafficked and 'marketed'. Biemann suggests that the Thai sex industry is being aided by the provision of migrant women from Cambodia, Laos and Vietnam, many of whom are 'lured with empty promises and smuggled across the borders into closed brothels or debt-bonded and condemned to do unpaid sex work for the trafficking ring for many years' (Biemann 2002: 77). This is as true for children as for adults, ethnic hill tribe children being trafficked into the country but also from the north to the beach resorts frequented by sex tourists.

What monitoring and interventions are undertaken to address these problems? In the US there is an annual assessment of each country's efforts to combat trafficking, known as TIPS (Trafficking in Persons). In the UK the Home Office Human Trafficking Centre (UKHTC) works to prevent trafficking, prosecute traffickers, and coordinate care to victims; reference was made in Chapter 5 to the pressure group ECPAT (www.ecpat.org.uk).

The health and health care of refugees

If people are forced to move they may be displaced across international borders, as refugees, or within the borders of their own countries, as 'internally displaced persons' (IDPs). A refugee is someone who seeks refuge, in a country other than that of their nationality, because of a fear of persecution due to their beliefs, or membership of a particular political or social group. In seeking refuge the person is said to be seeking asylum; protection afforded by a different nation state.

Evidence suggests that while the number of refugees has fallen since 1990 the number of IDPs has increased, notably in sub-Saharan Africa (Kalipeni and Oppong 1998, Roberts and Patel, 2010); The UNHCR (2010) suggests that in 2009 there were 43.3 million people across the globe forcibly displaced by conflict; of these, 27.1 million were IDPs. Pakistan, Iran and Syria were each host to over 1 million refugees, with the US and UK hosting 275,000 and 270,000 respectively. When one takes into account the economic capacity of the host country to manage refugee populations the relative burdens are very unequal and fall overwhelmingly on the least developed countries. Afghanistan accounted for one in four refugees (a total of 2.9 million), distributed across 71 countries (though the vast majority, 96%, found refuge in Pakistan), and Iraq almost 1.8 million. In addition to these vast numbers, the UN Office for the Coordination of Humanitarian Affairs suggests that at least 36 million people were displaced by natural disasters during 2008.

As Grove and Zwi (2006) assert, most displaced persons remain within the same region and only a small minority seek to settle in the global north. Despite this, the common perception is that countries in the developed world are being 'swamped' (a typical metaphor) by undeserving refugees. Ingram (2008) has charted in some detail the reactions of the popular press to health service access in the UK. A favourite theme is that of the 'scrounger' or undeserving asylum seeker 'jumping' NHS queues. As one newspaper (the Daily Star) advised its readers: 'good luck getting that appointment – remember every Algerian terrorist has the right to treatment before you'! (Ingram 2008: 884-5). This kind of reporting seriously downplays the risks faced in seeking a better place to live; for example, it is estimated that well over 1000 would-be migrants drown each year in making the Mediterranean crossing from North Africa to Italy on grossly overcrowded boats. At least 28 people died in December 2010 when a boat carrying Iraqis and Iranians crashed on rocks on Christmas Island – where Australia has an immigration detention centre. A BBC correspondent, Nick Bryant, reported that: 'With such harrowing images from Christmas Island broadcast on early evening news shows, millions of Australians would have seen the anguished faces of those seeking to reach its shores, and witnessed the lengths to which they would go to get there. Put simply, it was shockingly real. Tabloid sensationalism in Australia is normally turned against the asylum seekers. The disaster has already escalated the boat people debate...whatever its outcome, after the tragedy on Christmas Island the debate has a human face' (BBC website, 16 December 2010).

Grove and Zwi (2006) have illustrated how forced migrants are 'othered'; constructed, stigmatised and distanced as the deviant 'them' rather than the normal 'us'. The contemporary demonisation of those who would settle elsewhere brings to mind the reactions of those seeking, over the last five hundred years, to keep at bay and quarantine people thought to carry disease. The barbed wire and high walls of detention centres are the modern equivalents of the off-shore islands and moored ships that housed previous generations of would-be immigrants and pilgrims (see Chapter 8). The emphasis is less on the protection *of* the refugee and more the protection of the host population *from* the refugee (Grove and Zwi 2006). Such protection of the refugees as there is may only be temporary, leading to insecurity and anxiety about family members left behind who may be at risk of persecution.

Watters (2007) has set his discussion of refugees in Europe within the context of the 'moral economy of care', a context that reflects social values concerning what is legitimate and what is not; here, who is deserving of care and who is not. As in industrialised countries outside Europe a distinction is drawn between the 'genuine' refugee and those considered not genuine, variously labelled illegal immigrants, undocumented migrants, and bogus asylum seekers. From a geographical point of view the difficulty a refugee has in crossing a border is directly related to the differing wealth of the two countries; 'the proximity of an EU member state's border to countries with widely differing levels of GDP gives rise to the emergence of an enhanced security apparatus aimed at keeping people out' (Watters 2007: 400). In contrast, internal borders within the EU have been loosened.

The reality of the situation is illustrated by Watters' description of the Sangatte refugee camp near Calais in northern France. This was opened in 1999 by the Red Cross who realised that the only objective of those who arrived there (mostly young men from Africa) was to reach the UK. Some 68,000 migrants are thought to have lodged at the camp during its existence. Other would-be immigrants sought to enter the UK via the Belgian port of Zeebrugge, sadly well-known for the discovery of 58 Chinese migrants found dead in the back of a lorry in 2000. Many of those using Zeebrugge were very young (Watters suggests 90% were 15-18 years of age) and quite desperate to reach the UK. Even when they did arrive undetected they had little idea of what to do, lacking food and money and having little or no knowledge of the language. One can only wonder what the response of unsympathetic media commentators would be to desperate British adolescents forced to leave Europe for the safety of, say, China.

What health problems do refugees present to health services? These lie primarily in the area of chronic medical conditions. In their study of the ill-health of asylum seekers in Switzerland (primarily from the former Yugoslavia) Bischoff et al. (2009) found that the problems were due to musculoskeletal diseases, respiratory diseases, and poor mental health. As others have suggested, what this group requires is some continuity of care to deal with problems they have encountered in their mobile lives. Yet the focus tends to be on the risks, posed by refugees and asylum seekers, of spreading communicable disease. So just what are the consequences of forced migration for the spread of such disease?

Kazmi and Pandit (2001) sought to answer this question in the context of the movements of Afghan refugees into the North West Frontier Province of Pakistan, between 1972 and 1997.

They illustrate the considerable impact that the movements of over 2.5 million such refugees have had on the incidence of malaria. This arises because standing water in refugee camps provides a suitable breeding ground for the mosquitoes that carry the malaria parasite. In addition, exhausted and malnourished refugees had weakened immunity (and many arrived already infected with malaria) and were vulnerable to the disease. Careful mapping of changing incidence of the disease by district revealed a degree of spatial coincidence with the concentration of refugees.

Acknowledging the serious impediments to marshalling research evidence, Roberts and Patel (2010) have argued that forced migration increases vulnerability to HIV infection. The poverty that results from forced migration may lead to people exchanging unprotected sex (perhaps with local populations or in camps, or even aid workers) for money. Sexual violence perpetrated by soldiers is a depressing consequence of conflict and displacement, with appalling reports from recent conflicts in Sierra Leone and the Democratic Republic of the Congo, as well as former conflicts in Rwanda in the 1990s (Kalipeni and Oppong 1998: 1647). If, as some evidence suggests, armed combatants in these countries have above-average rates of HIV infection, the infection is likely to diffuse among the displaced population. But Roberts and Patel (2010) caution that in some cases forced migration might actually protect against such infection, especially if IDPs are 'housed' in camps that have relatively good provision of HIV/AIDS services. Regardless, we should be alert to attempts to stigmatise IDPs and refugees as inevitable disease vectors.

In an important paper focusing on African refugees Kalipeni and Oppong (1998) stress the need to set the associations between forced migration and disease into a broader, political ecology, context. The departure from previously farmed land can create food shortages and malnutrition if land is degraded, while healthcare that might have been available is perhaps no longer so – thereby lowering rates of immunisation and ante-natal care. These broader contextual factors can all lead to increased disease. Internal conflict in Mozambique in the 1980s destroyed almost half the country's health centres, as well as many schools and water supplies. Water supplies that do remain may be contaminated. Thus, while deaths and injury due directly to military activity are of course significant, many more are caused by the indirect consequences of war; namely, hunger and disease.

In south-east Asia a particular concern has been the displacement of people from the Shan ethnic group in eastern Burma, across the border in Thailand. Suwanvanichkij (2008) paints a grim picture of the forced relocation (ethnic cleansing, in effect), by the Burmese military (*Tatmadaw*), of several hundred thousand villagers over the last 15 years. With no official refugee camps in Thailand they become 'economic migrants' with few rights, tolerating abusive and exploitative working conditions merely because these are better than in Burma. As observed elsewhere, this displacement deprives them of access to basic health care, with the result that infectious diseases such as TB have become prevalent. Further, women forced by circumstances into the Thai sex industry are less likely to use condoms and Suwanvanichkij therefore speaks of a maturing epidemic of HIV/AIDS. He also refers to the displacement of Shan peoples as a result of dam construction on the Salween River, suggesting that displacement is a mix of both 'development' and political victimisation.

With particular reference to HIV/AIDS Anderson (2010) notes the problems faced in accessing health care for those seeking asylum, particularly when they are labelled as undeserving by the popular press (see also Ingram 2008, who quotes a 2001 headline from the right-wing paper the *Daily Mail*: 'AIDS epidemic fear as thousands of African victims pour into the UK'). As Anderson notes, 'being both an asylum applicant and living with HIV means carrying a doubly compromised social identity' (Anderson 2010: 81). Those whose applications fail face the risk of being returned to countries that have poor provision of care for those with infectious disease, while many migrants present later for HIV services than do the native-born population and fail to reap benefits from anti-retroviral agents.

Those forced to move are therefore exposed to new infections or expose others to infections they bring with them. Malnutrition weakens immune systems and puts refugees at further risk. Cholera epidemics (see Chapter 8) have long been a feature of refugee movements; some 50,000 Rwandan refugees are thought to have died in refugee camps as a result of cholera and dysentery (Aagaard-Hansen et al. 2010). Refugees forced by conflict in Afghanistan into refugee camps in Pakistan are also exposed to neglected tropical diseases such as schistosomiasis and leishmaniasis.

The mental health consequences of forced displacement due to conflict are potentially devastating. Exposure to war and violence – at worst, witnessing close family members killed or maimed – is acutely traumatic, as stories of Cambodians escaping the brutal Khmer Rouge regime can only begin to convey (Kemp and Rasbridge 2004: 39). UNICEF suggested that among unaccompanied children in Sudan in 1993 almost all had been shot at, or witnessed killings, or had lost a close family member (Kalipeni and Oppong 1998: 1648). The forced displacement is itself traumatic, as is the separation of family members. UNICEF estimated that some 114,000 children were separated from their families during the Rwandan conflict (Kalipeni and Oppong 1998: 1648).

As a marker of the most severe consequences for mental health some researchers have turned to epidemiological studies using measures of post-traumatic stress. Several studies have looked at post-conflict populations in parts of Africa. Onyut et al. (2009) examined the prevalence of post-traumatic stress disorder (PTSD) and depression among over 1400 refugees who had fled Somalia and Rwanda for Uganda. Nearly one-third of those from Rwanda, and about a half of the Somali refugees living in an official refugee settlement, were deemed to have PTSD. Three-quarters had witnessed dead or mutilated bodies, 60% had seen beatings or torture, and 51% had witnessed people killed. All this was compounded by poor physical health and poor nutrition. Consequently, the health care needs are many, but include greater attention to mental health interventions. Also in Africa, Roberts and colleagues (2009) looked at PTSD and depression among 1200 adults, most of whom had been displaced to Juba in southern Sudan as a result of conflict lasting 20 years. Over a third of this sample (but more women than men) had symptoms of PTSD and half were diagnosed with depression. These problems endure. For example, Ehntholt and Yule (2006) report on a follow-up study of 40 adolescent Cambodian refugees, half of whom suffered PTSD and depression four years after leaving Cambodia, rates that had dropped only to 35% twelve years later.

In a different geo-political context, and in a study undertaken by Médecins Sans Frontières, de Jong and colleagues (2007) looked at the psychosocial health of those displaced by the conflict in Chechnya, both within the republic of Chechnya but also in neighbouring Ingushetia. Almost one-quarter of the 650 people interviewed had witnessed killings, and half had observed maltreatment. Over three-quarters reported suffering from depression or social dysfunction. Of course, this rather sanitised epidemiological study (like others discussed above) does not begin to convey the real experience; as de Jong and colleagues put it, it is 'incorrect to reduce the experience of conflict and violence to the individual using bio-psycho-medical terminology'. Research conducted within a positivist framework, that presupposes mental illness can be assessed using standardised questionnaire 'instruments', contrasts with more constructionist perspectives which suggest that mental health varies across cultural groups and that a Western clinical approach is not necessarily appropriate.

The mental health impacts outlined above can be thought of as the direct effects of conflict and associated forced migration. Indirect effects that result from the dislocation and seeking asylum include the lack of employment and good housing, frequent changes in accommodation, and lengthy delays in having asylum applications processed. Linked to the latter is the stress of uncertainty over the application and the prospect of being deported. All these contribute to serious psychological problems, including depression and anxiety. But generalisation is dangerous; outcomes depend on the politico-geographic context from which those displaced have sought refuge, and the extent of welcome or otherwise they face in a host country.

The issue of frequent changes of address is highlighted in a study of Somali refugees in London (Warfa et al. 2006). Using in-depth interviews and focus groups an erratic pattern of movement across east London is traced; refugees move from one deprived area to another, including across health care administrative boundaries, meaning that the agencies responsible for care will be different. Consider one person's experience: 'When I came to this country I was taken to a hostel in London. After a while I moved to a friend's house but could not live there and started looking for another hostel in Hammersmith. I then moved to Bristol looking for a job and stayed there for a while and came back to London and lived in Southall. I moved to Manchester and eventually settled in Leicester. After three years I returned back to London...' (in Warfa et al. 2006: 508). Clearly, this is a chaotic existence, made more difficult by poor housing conditions and poor employment opportunities. The frequent moves have detrimental effects on mental health; the popular notion of a nomadic Somali existence that some would use to explain their predilection for mobility is certainly not confirmed in this study.

While work such as this in the UK suggests chaotic lives and poor mental health, treatment of refugees in some parts of the 'developed' world is worse. In Australia, for example, immigration detention centres (IDCs) are part of a hard-line treatment of those seeking asylum (McLoughlin and Warin 2008), a perspective that developed alongside concerns that the country would be 'swamped' by 'boat people' arriving from south-east Asia in the 1980s and 1990s. IDCs therefore hold any undocumented arrival, pending a decision on their status, a decision that can take up to seven years. The locations themselves are isolated, including in remote coastal or arid regions, and the centres are surrounded by razor wire and heavily controlled by security guards; effectively, they are prisons. There is plenty of evidence (reviewed by McLoughlin and Warin) that IDCs erode the lives of those incarcerated therein, adding to mental health burdens. As one detainee put it: 'I was carrying a mountain of burdens when I came seeking hope, seeing asylum in Australia. Unfortunately, upon my arrival, my burdens increased and my suffering led me to a new state of madness in Australia' (cited in McLoughlin and Warin 2008: 260). In response to criticisms the Australian government has recently been reviewing its policy on detention.

What can be done to mitigate the poor state of mental health and well-being endured by refugees? Obvious though it may seem, an understanding of the cultural, as well as traumatic physical, displacement is required. There is 'cultural bereavement' in leaving one country and settling in another and thereby being forced to straddle two cultures; the one left behind and the one in that host country (Crowley 2009). From a clinical perspective Ehntholt and Yule (2006) suggest that therapy needs to establish safety and trust but that psychological and psychiatric interventions need to be allied with knowledge of immigration law. Cognitive-behavioural therapy (CBT) has been shown to work with children and adolescents, as well as adults who have been victims of torture. Other interventions, such as nurse-led clinics in hostels, specialist health visitors, link workers and translators can all play a part, though one has to question whether these services will remain in place as western countries slash public sector expenditure. But mental health problems do not necessarily arise; some children and adolescents prove remarkably resilient and cope with a new environment (Crowley 2009). In addition, what may be needed to address mental health problems is less of a clinical focus and more a recognition that better housing, good education, decent job opportunities, and less discrimination are what are required. Again, however, such resources may be in short supply in times of economic downturn.

Sampson and Gifford (2010) draw on classic geographic ideas to suggest that, in Melbourne, Australia, young refugees develop strategies to actively seek out and benefit from places that promote healing and recovery. They link this to ideas of 'reterritorialisation' – the creation of new spaces (or therapeutic landscapes) to counter the 'deterritorialisation' that accompanies the loss of attachment to the former home. Young people aged 11-19 years, primarily from Sudan, Iraq and Ethiopia, used visual methods (such as photographs and sketches of neighbourhoods) to identify places they felt important to them and liked, as well as those they disliked. Schools, parks and libraries featured high on the list of places of welcome, offering possibilities for developing new social relationships, while green spaces were regarded as places of restoration. Of course, we should not over-romanticise this; for many refugees the experience of new places is quite traumatic, given the social and physical isolation that those not at school or at work can feel. Places marked with offensive graffiti, or unfamiliar busy roads, are threatening rather than therapeutic.

Development and disaster

Adey (2010: 115-6) notes that major development projects (such as the construction of dams) in the global south have displaced huge numbers of people, though smaller-scale projects (road construction, mining projects) are at least as significant. Lerer and Scudder (1999: 114) suggest that dams are a 'paradigm for globalization in poorer countries'. In India up to 38 million people have been displaced by large dam construction projects undertaken to improve water supply and irrigation. The displacements are patterned socially, with the politically weak and marginalised powerless to object. The benefits are not necessarily reaped locally; rather, the electricity flows to the major centres of industry and population.

The health consequences of this kind of displacement are unlikely to be as severe as those of refugees displaced by political conflict and war. Nonetheless, there are serious consequences for economic status and psychological well-being. The indirect consequences are much the same as portrayed by Kalipeni and Oppong (1998) in their study of African refugees; loss and degradation of land and housing; dismantling of family and social networks; and food insecurity. All these will contribute to increased morbidity and mortality as people are physically displaced. The influx of construction workers brings further risks of infectious disease transmission and of accidents (Lerer and Scudder 1999).

Among the most well-known dam projects is the Kariba Dam on the Zambezi River separating Zimbabwe and Zambia. Built in the late 1950s it displaced over 100,000 people from land that subsequently became degraded; those affected showed increased incidence of diseases such as measles, dysentery and sleeping sickness soon after resettlement (Robinson, 2002: 54). Robinson (2002: 48-9) reports official statistics that over 10 million Chinese were displaced by dam-building projects between 1950 and 1990, while significant numbers have been displaced by the Three Gorges Dam (completed in 2009) on the Yangtze River. Cao, Hwang and Xi (2008) suggest that over 1.3 million have been displaced (with over 26 thousand hectares of land flooded) and they have examined the health consequences of constructing the dam, using data collected from a sample of several hundred migrants and non-migrants, both before and after relocation. Their results, which focus on psycho-social health, show evidence of significant health differences between the two cohorts. Dam construction has affected the health of migrants directly but also indirectly via social changes to community life and reductions in household income.

'Natural' disasters (such as earthquakes, tsunamis, floods, and extreme weather events) can occur in much the same geographic areas, and at much the same time, as political conflict. As Spiegel and his colleagues (2007) note, the Asian tsunami in 2004 that killed over 280,000 people and devastated Aceh Province in Indonesia and part of the coast of Sri Lanka affected areas that were the focus of rebel insurgencies, while drought in the Horn of Africa goes hand in hand with political conflict. I put 'natural' in inverted commas to suggest that, while disasters may have an origin in geophysical or atmospheric conditions, their consequences are often exacerbated by human – and particularly governmental – responses. Poor maintenance of infrastructure, poor coordination of evacuation, and apparent official indifference all turn a natural disaster into a hybrid of the social and the natural.

I want here to comment on the health consequences of such disasters, including the resulting disruption. It might be imagined that the spread of infectious disease is a primary risk, but there is little evidence that epidemics of infectious disease are a common consequence of large-scale natural disasters, despite frequent assertions to the contrary (Spiegel et al. 2007). It might also be thought that high rates of mortality go hand-in-hand with such disasters. While this is of course sometimes the case, as noted above, there are other, more enduring impacts.

As noted in Bourque et al. (2006) hurricanes in the Caribbean and Gulf States of the US are nothing new, and they trace the impact that each has had in the region since 1985. But in late August 2005 much of New Orleans was devastated by Hurricane Katrina. More than 1100 people were killed in Louisiana, and about 350 in other Gulf coast states (Jonkman et al. 2009). Most of the fatalities were older adults (85% were older than 50 years of age), suggesting a difficulty or unwillingness to be evacuated before the hurricane arrived. Although 55% of the deaths were African Americans, Jonkman et al. (2009) suggest this is in proportion to the distribution within the affected population; there is no evidence that African Americans were more likely to have died. While many deaths were due directly to drowning, deaths that occurred among evacuees were related to the stress of the move or to under-provision of health services.

Some estimates (Jonkman et al. 2009: 678) suggest that 1.1 million people (in almost half a million vehicles) evacuated the New Orleans region before the storm arrived. Many of the 72,000 who remained after evacuation found their way to the main sports stadium (the Superdome), where conditions rapidly deteriorated. Adey (2010: 86-7) and Cresswell (2006: Epilogue) have discussed in more detail the social dimension of evacuation. Adey comments that 'the evacuation plan for the city was predicated on an assumption of unified access to private transportation' (Adey 2010: 86); but some 250,000 residents had no private transport, and the 464 available buses were only ever going to evacuate 10% of that population (Bourque et al. 2006). While only 5% of the white population lacked access to a car, 27% of the African American population lacked such access; Adey refers to 'a clear racial politics of access'. For poor black people rapid evacuation along the highways, in a private car, was not an option, and those immobilised were the most vulnerable. As Cresswell (2006: 262) expresses it, 'mobility is social through and through'.

He also reminds us that media descriptions of those displaced as 'refugees' were objected to by others, who presumably felt this term was not appropriate for Americans since it bracketed them with 'other' (foreign and suspect) refugees, a class apart one presumes.

A number of post-disaster studies have been conducted to gauge the extent of the human impact. The Centers for Disease Control (CDC) conducted an assessment of needs seven weeks after the event, interviewing residents in two areas of New Orleans (MMWR 2006). In one, Orleans Parish (where median income was $27,000 compared with $42,000 for the US as a whole), the results suggested considerable disruption and impact (Table 6.1). These include: few utilities and services; substantial damage to property; and problems obtaining medical care. In addition, while a high proportion of the sample reported pre-existing chronic illness, almost half had become ill since the flooding.

Table 6.1   **Percentage of homes with health-related consequences reported in October 2005 after Hurricane Katrina (August 2005); Orleans Parish**

Consequences	Percentage
No electricity	65.5
No running water	53.8
No working toilet	57.9
No garbage removal	69.8
Severe damage to property	42.7
Problems obtaining medical care	32.9
Pre-existing chronic illness	60.4
Illness since hurricane	41.3

Source: MMWR (2006: 41)

Other surveys in New Orleans indicated that 43% of people felt isolated. Adams et al. (2009: 619) report that within six months of the disaster there had been more than 90,000 counselling sessions and 13,000 referrals for mental health services. In part, this will have been because people waited for lengthy periods without knowing what had happened to family members (Bourque et al. 2006). A fortnight after the hurricane struck almost a half of those evacuated to Houston said that they were still seeking family members or friends. A more detailed study of over 1000 displaced households (Abramson et al. 2008) conducted face-to-face interviews both 6-12 months, and then 20-23 months, after the disaster. At both periods, more than half the respondents reported significant mental health problems, particularly if there were children in the household and social networks had been disrupted. Writing four years after the event Adams et al. (2009) suggest that those who were displaced suffer from 'chronic disaster syndrome', by which they mean not solely the individual psychological effects but also the wider set of structural determinants that place such people at relative disadvantage. The personal trauma, the disrupted social networks, and the relocation of impoverished people combine to create a nexus of misfortune. 'Families fell apart not simply because they were dispersed to places far distant, but because [they lacked] the physical and emotional structure of routines holding people in place' (Adams et al. 2009: 623). And the government let private companies, including those working in the security industry, take lucrative contracts that replaced the social welfare and public sector investment that had characterised pre-Katrina New Orleans.

Adams and colleagues' (2009) account is worth reading for the detailed stories told by a set of 180 displaced residents. They use these stories to paint a picture of how the poor were evicted. 'They were uprooted and sent to a prison camp of a trailer park hours outside the city and with no access to public transportation, jobs, stores, clinics, and schools. And then, with no place to return to in the city, they were told to vacate the trailers they had been sent to' (Adams et al. 2009: 628). In a telling phrase, people spoke about having lost the 'ingredients of life'. Two years after the disaster, shops were still boarded up, roads were full of cracks and pot-holes, and many were awaiting insurance company claims to be settled.

Displacement, then, is highly structured socially, with those who are relatively well-off having a very different mobility 'experience' from those who are poor (Grieco and Hine 2008). An understanding of this experience is incomplete without recognising the economic and political context that seeks to aid recovery but often slows it down. Bourque and colleagues (2006: 145) put it succinctly: 'Disasters enhance socially structured inequalities already in place'. For many, the disaster that was Katrina is chronic and ongoing.

Concluding remarks

The mobilities described here are very different from those encountered in much of the 'mobilities turn' literature. Some of the people we have encountered here speak to us of unimaginable experiences, completely different from those living in the western world. Not for them the frequent air travel, the pleasurable car trip, or the Mediterranean cruise; rather, the dangers of stowing away or risking life on an over-crowded boat.

What do the groups considered in this chapter have in common? While generalisation is difficult we could suggest that all are vulnerable; many are hidden from view in shadow economies; all are socially marginalised; and all find themselves in situations not of their own choosing but in circumstances in which wider social structures and organisations shape – at worst, control – their lives. If we are to address contemporary slavery, and to help those at risk of trafficking, if we are to give better assistance to those displaced by development or disaster, we surely need to attend more to the 'upstream' factors that determine individual life chances.

Chapter 7
Migration, Health and Well-being

Introduction

My aim in this chapter is to consider some of the relationships between migration, health and well-being, and access to healthcare. Migration can be voluntary or involuntary (forced) and I considered the health impacts of the latter in the previous chapter. My focus here is on the reflexive relationship between voluntary migration and health. Migration can have an impact on the mover's health, while the mover's health status will affect her or his propensity to migrate. Examining these relationships has spawned a large literature.

I want here to consider the following sets of issues. First, I shall say something about the process of migration itself, the laying down of roots in a new environment, and the impacts on mental health and well-being. Next, I consider differences between movers and non-movers and in particular the 'selectivity' of migration; the fact that movers are not a random sub-set of the population as a whole. I then turn to the longer-term impacts of migration and health – issues of acculturation and adaptation. Last, I consider one particular aspect of the impact of migration on the health of communities. This is 'population mixing'; the possibility that, as host populations become exposed to new infections as a result of in-migration, rare diseases such as childhood leukaemia may increase in incidence.

There is a wealth of studies that reveal how mortality differs according to country of birth. This analysis relies on linking mortality and population census data. For example, in England and Wales Wild and colleagues (2007) showed that standardised mortality ratios (all-causes) were significantly elevated among the following groups: men born in Bangladesh; women born in India or Pakistan; and both men and women born in West Africa. Young men (20-44 years) born in Eastern Europe were also at high risk of death, particularly from heart disease.

But such studies tend to be under-theorised. Aside from speculating on possible 'lifestyle' influences (such as smoking and alcohol consumption) Wild's study is light on explanation. Nonetheless, this sort of study provides a context for what follows in this chapter.

Migration and mental health

I first assess the evidence concerning the impact of migration on mental health, at the individual and family level. In the main, I am concerned with international migration; while, as I showed earlier, the mental health impacts of forced migration may be many times more severe than for those whose moves are not forced upon them, there are consequences for the latter groups too.

Such impacts can be positive as well as negative. Migration offers, to the relatively disadvantaged in poor countries, the prospects of economic improvement, including the remittance of money to family members back home. But it can also be stressful, leading to mental health problems as people seek to come to terms with a new social and cultural environment. As well as having to 'adapt' to new norms, they may be faced with a hostile reception – most obviously, if they do not speak the host language or are of different colour. There may be problems of social isolation, particularly for women left at home while their male partners are at work; this was evidenced in Elliott and Gillie's study (1998) of Fijian migrant women in British Columbia, Canada. Such women struggled to maintain cultural traditions and felt quite homesick.

The associations between discrimination and racism, and the health of ethnic minorities, including immigrants, has been a focus of recent investigation. Discrimination against, and harassment of, immigrant groups, is associated with poor health (Karlsen and Nazroo 2002). Immigrants to Spain from Ecuador, Colombia, Morocco and Romania, for example, reported experiences of racism and poor working conditions, as well as being limited in terms of employment opportunities; such discrimination affects mental health (Agudelo-Suárez et al. 2009). Interestingly, there seems to be a 'pecking order' of 'acceptability'. As one Colombian woman puts it: 'Colombians here in Spain get a positive reaction in comparison with Romanians, Arabs, Algerians; we could say that we are not viewed badly or mistreated in comparison, but in comparison with other nationalities we are discriminated against, for example they appreciate people from Argentina better than Colombians' (Agudelo-Suárez et al. 2009: 1870).

The move itself may be quite stressful, and this will be magnified for those travelling long distances and particularly from one country to another. Anyone who has relocated even a short distance can attest to the stress involved in making the purchase and overseeing the move. Any move involves some social dislocation and fracturing of relationships that may be difficult to maintain post-migration. This sense of dislocation may, for some, be the precursor to later mental health problems – and physical health problems too. As Ott and her colleagues (2008: 525) note, 'continuous exposure to high stress levels can cause a central nervous system and endocrine response, which itself may increase the risk for cardiovascular (CVD) and suicide mortality'.

There is substantial evidence of an increased risk of suicide among migrants. We have known since Durkheim's classic early 20th century study that isolation and lack of integration are risk factors. Ott and colleagues looked at a cohort of nearly 35,000 immigrants from the former Soviet Union to Germany and followed this group to determine mortality risk from various causes. Male immigrants had a markedly higher risk of suicide than native-born Germans; the risk was highest shortly after a move. Again, problems of integration seem to arise. Suicide risk seems to vary with country of origin. For example (Lindert et al. 2008), immigrants to Germany from Turkey and Morocco seem to be at lower risk than those from Surinam. These differences may possibly be explained by religious belief and levels of within-group cohesion. The link between residential mobility and suicide risk does not seem solely to apply to international migrants. A study in Texas cited by Ott and her colleagues found that change of address within the last 12 months led to a doubling of the risk of attempted suicide compared with those who had not moved; the explanation lay in poor job prospects and lack of social support.

Some researchers have looked at other suicide 'behaviour', which encompasses thoughts ('ideation') about suicide, and attempts at taking one's life. While this may apply to migrants it also appears to apply to the children of migrants, who may have difficulty fitting in to a cultural setting in which they are a minority. Thus van Bergen and colleagues (2008) observed that adolescents of Turkish background living in the Netherlands were significantly more likely than other adolescents to consider suicide. This is ascribed to poor self-image and anxieties about not becoming successful in life; it does not appear to simply reflect socio-economic circumstances. Moreover, suicide risk appears to be elevated among family members left behind when others migrate. Borges and his colleagues (2008) found that families of those migrating from Mexico to the US were at greater risk of suicidal ideation and attempt than Mexicans who did not migrate. This suggests there are other stresses – those associated with the disruption of family networks.

In relation to serious mental health problems there is long-standing interest in the association between migration and schizophrenia. Cantor-Graae and Selten (2005) have provided a meta-analysis of the literature. This pooling of a large number of studies reveals that there is a genuine association; migrants seem to be three times as likely as non-migrants to develop schizophrenia, and those from the global south seem to be at greater risk than those from elsewhere. The explanation is not wholly clear but 'the long-term experience of social defeat, i.e. the chronic stressful experience of outsider status' (Cantor-Graae and Selten 2005: 21) is a plausible explanation.

It may well be that socio-economic status confounds the possible association between migration and (mental) health status. In other words, do migrants show worse (mental) health than others because they are poorer or from more deprived backgrounds? For sure, in many cases they will have low rates of participation in labour markets and therefore lower levels of income. Some studies (Lindert et al. 2008) suggest that the mental health of migrants from Mexico to the US worsens with length of stay; this might be due to discrimination, or lack of job opportunities, or perhaps failed expectations.

A relatively under-researched area is the relationship between migration and mental health in older populations. The motivation for migration of older adults may centre on life events such as retirement or loss of a partner, or declining health. Such life events can be stressful and trigger migration; both the events and the move may contribute to depressive symptoms, with 'negative' events perhaps more likely to contribute to psychological ill-health than others, and women likely to be worse affected than men. However, empirical work by Bradley and van Willigen (2010) in the US suggests that migration might be therapeutic for recently bereaved women, perhaps because they move closer to other family members who can offer support. And any negative impacts on health may not be long-lasting; the psychological impact of the move lessens once the initial stresses are overcome and migrants become used to their new environment, establishing new social networks or re-establishing former ones (Bradley and van Willigen 2010: 7). This research clearly emphasises the importance of social support and integration – the maintenance or development of social capital to set alongside the 'mobility capital' expressed in the move itself perhaps.

Relatively little research has examined changes to mental health after migration from one non-western country to another. Anbesse and colleagues (2009) have undertaken qualitative research to explore the experiences of female domestic servants from Ethiopia, working in four Middle Eastern countries. All had returned to Ethiopia, some with serious mental health problems. Regardless of mental health status, themes of inhumane treatment, the undermining of cultural identity and enforced cultural isolation emerged from interviews. Some women spoke of being exhausted and overwhelmed by work demands, and themselves linked this to the development of mental ill-health (Anbesse et al. 2009: 560). As one put it, the employers 'don't see you as a human being', while for another 'they see us like as if we are slaves'. Abu-habib (1998) studied female domestic workers from Sri Lanka migrating to Lebanon, migration encouraged by the Sri Lankan government because of the income accruing from wages sent home; but these economic benefits were countered by lack of job security or benefits or employment protection, and by the stigma faced by such women when they returned home.

In these and other studies the notion of migration as simply a relocation from one place to another is clearly impoverished. There is *dis*location, a social as well as spatial separation, with the migrants' lives and new social worlds tightly controlled. The *international migration* may have been voluntary, but the *local movements* and opportunities for social interaction once ensconced in a new country can be highly restricted.

What difficulties in accessing health care are faced by those migrating voluntarily? If, as we see below, immigrants tend over time to lose their health advantage over native-born populations, a question is whether this is due to their relatively poorer access to health care. A number of studies in North America have addressed this, and are reviewed in Lebrun and Dubay (2010). These suggest that in the US, compared with the native-born, immigrants are less likely to have health insurance. Undocumented immigrants get no health insurance and even legal immigrants are not eligible for federally funded health insurance until they have lived in the country for five years. Immigrant women may not be adequately screened for cervical and breast cancer. In Canada immigrants have fewer consultations with physicians and, again, less access to screening. Yet it is too simple to say that immigrants have poorer access than native-born; once adjustment for socio-economic and demographic status is made there is relatively little effect of place of birth on health care usage.

Immigrants in the US have low levels of health insurance in part because some are employed in workplaces that do not provide such insurance, in part because they may not be able to afford private medical insurance but also because there are restrictions on access of immigrants to Medicaid (Fennelly 2007). The RAND Corporation estimates that undocumented adult immigrants – who comprise about 3% of the population – account for only 1.5% of US medical costs (Okie 2007). Of course, this under-utilisation may only in part reflect lack of need; more likely it reflects an unwillingness to be exposed to scrutiny. Fennelly (2007) suggests that it is a myth that immigrants consume substantial volumes of scarce healthcare resources. She argues that, in the US, per capita expenditure on healthcare for immigrants was only 45% of that for US-born people. This is because they have lower levels of obesity and cardiovascular disease. There is also evidence of late presentation to clinics among immigrant groups, a feature that is unlikely to confer health benefits on them. Immigrants may also lack access to screening programmes, whether for infectious disease or cancer. This may reflect language barriers, but the lack of resources needed to secure treatment is likely to figure more prominently.

Chakrabati (2010) has shown how 'care' can be delivered to immigrants not merely locally but also 'at a distance'. Drawing on interviews with 40 pregnant Bengali immigrant women in New York City she reveals that the social networks on which the women rely are often transnational. With the increasing availability of new communication technologies, as well as traditional ones ('phone cards have become like medicine', as one of her respondents puts it), contact is retained with family and friends in Bangladesh, the latter offering all kinds of advice (on nutrition in particular). More locally in neighbourhoods, advice on foodstuffs, as well as the exchange of food itself, proved sustaining socially as well as physically. Chakrabati calls these networks 'social therapeutic networks', and in doing so extends health geographers' classic engagement with 'therapeutic landscapes' to embed social networks into that framework. I discuss social networking more fully in Chapter 10.

The selectivity of migration

Migrants are not a random sub-set of the population, and the social and demographic characteristics of migrants are likely to be quite different from those of non-movers (Boyle and Norman 2010). They differ in terms of age, educational attainment, and socio-economic and health status. As a result, we can speak of the 'selectivity' of migration and I need to say something about the health consequences of this (see Fennelly 2007, for an overview).

There are three broad sets of studies of migrant health (Cunningham et al. 2008). We might contrast the health of a migrant population (those from a particular country or racial/ethnic group) with that of the new host population. Second, we can compare the health of migrants with the health of those born in the host country but of the same sub-group. Last, we might assess the health of the migrants with that of those remaining behind. In all cases there is a mix of evidence; in some cases migrants seem to do better than non-migrants, but in other cases they do worse. Much depends on where they relocate. Cunningham and colleagues (2008) review evidence on the health of foreign-born people in the US and suggest that most studies report lower mortality rates among foreign-born compared with native-born Americans, as well as lower incidence of heart disease. Women born overseas seem to have reduced risk of low birth-weight babies compared to US-born women. In addition, immigrants from some countries in Asia show a 10-year advantage in life expectancy compared with the average in the sending countries.

In a classic paper Graham Bentham (1988) looked in some detail at the relation between migration and health, noting that pre-retirement migration rates tend to be higher among young people employed in professional occupations. Since this demographic group tends to have better health than the population as a whole it may be that the loss of such people from particular areas can worsen the overall health profile of such areas (as well as perhaps improving the health of the destinations). This is important in view of the considerable interest in the geography of health inequalities. It is well-known (Gatrell and Elliott 2009) that there are strong relationships between area deprivation and mortality and ill-health. But migration may affect these relationships, and evidence that health inequalities in richer countries may be worsening over time could, in fact, be due to migration. In other words, the health gap between poor and wealthier areas could be explained as much by the selectivity of population movement, as by area deprivation. Work by Norman and his colleagues (2005) using English longitudinal data seems to support this; in the most deprived areas it is the outward movement of the relatively healthy, and the immobility of those who are less healthy, that appears to explain changing relationships between population health and deprivation.

Wen and colleagues (2010) have contrasted the health of migrants to Shanghai, China with that of 'urban natives'. Migrants appear to have higher levels of self-assessed health than do those native to Shanghai, and this finding is consistent with the health selection hypothesis of healthier individuals being 'self-selected' for migration. Lu (2008) has examined the health determinants of the migration decision in Indonesia. He confirms the selectivity of migration for those moving within the country. Younger people in good health are more likely to move than those who are not. Older people in poor health tend to migrate to join other family members or to seek improved health care, or to relocate to retirement destinations that are perceived to be better for their health. Bentham (1988) demonstrated that, in the UK, migration of older adults tends to be selective of those in poor health moving shorter distances, perhaps to be closer to care settings. Larson and her colleagues (2004) confirmed this for Australian women aged 45-50 years; both short-distance and long-distance moves within the country were associated with chronic poor health. As they express it, 'it is time to put aside the myth of the healthy migrant who boldly moves to maximise his or her economic and social gains within national boundaries. While the characterisation may be true for young people, the weight of evidence suggests that it is not true of mature adults' (Larson et al. 2004: 2158). Like other research, this study is based on the analysis of large data-sets and there is a need for more qualitative research to help explain migration processes among different age groups.

Migration, then, appears to be selective of those with better health. But why this selectivity? As implied above, many will be moving for employment reasons and, if employed, they are likely to be in better health than those who are not, since they may have physically or intellectually demanding jobs to go to. Equally, those in employment are more likely to be able to bear the costs – financial and personal – involved in migrating. Those with poorer health may be less likely to migrate because of the physical upheaval and mental stress involved with the move.

It is important to reinforce that the relationship between health status and migration depends on context, especially across the life course. While mobile young adults do indeed report better health than non-migrants, in older adulthood the pattern may be reversed, with the unhealthy more likely to move. In an interesting paper Tunstall and her colleagues (2010) have focused on a particular class of migrant, those women living in the UK who are either pregnant or are new mothers. They find that this group is an exception to the norm; they have poorer health than non-movers. This is less to do with mobility, they argue, and more a function of their lower socio-economic status; this in turn may be associated with family breakdown. Wiking and colleagues (2004) looked at samples of immigrants to Sweden from Poland, Iran and Turkey, comparing their self-reported health with that of Swedish-born men and women. Turkish and Iranian men were three times as likely as Swedish men to report poor health, with immigrant women from those countries five times as likely. But as with Tunstall's study the explanation seemed to lie in socio-economic status; in other words it is not being born overseas that matters so much as poor socio-economic status.

Health selectivity in migration may help to explain some of the differences between the population health of different groups. For example, given their relatively low socio-economic status one might expect Hispanics in the US to have worse health than the white population; in fact, they seem to have better health outcomes. This apparently surprising finding may be due to the selective migration of Hispanics into the US; the hypothesis is that Hispanics entering the US are healthier than those remaining behind. For example, Landale and her colleagues (2006) have shown that rates of infant mortality among women migrants from Puerto Rico to the US mainland are less than non-migrant women. However, as their length of residence in the US increases, so does the risk of infant mortality. Any benefits this group of Puerto Ricans may have enjoyed before arrival seem to dissipate with exposure to life on the mainland. This issue of assimilation is addressed in the next section.

Migration and acculturation

By acculturation is meant the extent to which immigrants 'adopt' the characteristics of the host population. A considerable literature has emerged that explores this, though the focus tends to be on the extent to which the individual assimilates, as if it were somehow solely their responsibility. As with so many aspects of social life, acculturation will be shaped both by the individual's agency and the location they find themselves occupying in social space.

Migrant health, and ability to adapt, is affected by place characteristics, such as exposure to polluted environments, and poor access to public amenities can play a part in shaping subsequent health. Depending on their material circumstances immigrants will often find themselves concentrated in areas of relative socio-economic deprivation. The question of whether these contextual factors matter has been explored by Lorant et al. (2008) in a study of the self-reported health of immigrants to Belgium from Morocco and Turkey. Over two-thirds of immigrants from those countries were, in 2001, living in the poorest areas of environmental quality, compared with 17% of native-born Belgians. But some spatial settings are protective. For example, the authors found that immigrant health was improved in areas with high concentrations of immigrant populations; there seems to be some form of protective effect, suggesting that ethnic concentration confers advantages, including the creation and maintenance of social networks and the integration of newly arrived immigrants (Lorant et al. 2008: 688). Further, social policy in respect of housing makes a difference; the authors contrast the housing stock on offer in Belgium with the poor blocks of suburban council flats that house immigrants in France, the focus of riots in 2005.

Viruell-Fuentes (2007) is critical of the rather individualistic, culturally-based notion of acculturation, claiming that, as a 'catch-all' construct it neglects the wider societal structural constraints which migrants face. Rather than perhaps blaming immigrants (in her study, Mexicans in the US) for not adapting more readily to new environments she points to their being treated poorly by the native-born. Thus it is not so much what she refers to as 'behavioral norm-swapping' that accounts for poor health; rather, it is deep-rooted attitudes towards 'others' (discrimination, put simply). This provides an explanation for the worsening health of Latino populations in the USA; those who migrated at a young age find, through the education system, that they have 'an acute sense of their ascribed social position in the US racial hierarchy, i.e. a minority position associated with economic, political, and social exclusion' (Viruell-Fuentes 2007: 1531).

Her qualitative research with Mexican immigrant women living in Southwest Detroit, Michigan suggests that first-generation immigrants (those born in Mexico and migrating to the US as adults) experienced less discrimination than those who moved as children or were born to first generation immigrants. A possible explanation is that the former moved into neighbourhoods that had high concentrations of Mexicans; these provided possibilities for the creation of social networks and protected women from exposure to possible stigmatisation. But as one 47 year old put it 'it's when your world meets the other world that there are clashes and problems' (Viruell-Fuentes 2007: 1529).

Let me now say something about the ways in which immigrants assume the behaviours and lifestyles of the host population. It is useful to know this as it provides evidence concerning the relative importance of genetic and environmental causes of disease. If, for instance, migrants from an area of low incidence of a chronic disease gradually show higher incidence after living some years in a new country, this would suggest some role for environmental factors.

There are many examples of this kind of study (see Gatrell and Elliott 2009: 163-6 for an overview). I focus on just one – obesity – since it is of course associated with 'mobility'. Further, since we know that obesity is associated with heart disease and stroke, as well as diabetes, and since the potential costs to health-care systems are considerable, it is of great public (health) concern. What evidence is there, then, that increased body weight is associated with immigration, or that it increases with length of residence?

There seems to be very consistent evidence of an 'acculturation' effect. Cairney and Ostbye (1999) showed that while the average body-mass index (BMI) for women born in Canada was 24.9 kg/m^2, women who had lived in Canada for less than five years had a BMI of only 22.7, but this rose to 24.8 for those who had lived in Canada for more than 10 years. In a cross-sectional study of a US sample of 32,000 participants (14% of whom were immigrants), Goel et al. (2004) found that while the prevalence of obesity was 16% among immigrants and 22% among the US-born, these proportions changed with length of residence. The prevalence was only 8% for those who had lived in the US for less than a year, but 19% for those who had lived there for more than 15 years. Kaplan and his colleagues (2004) have confirmed these findings in a study of Hispanic-born immigrants to the US. The prevalence of obesity among those with less than 5 years residence was just under 10%, but this rose to almost one-quarter (24.2%) among those with more than 15 years residence. Of course, much depends on context and country of origin. For example, the category 'Hispanic' can cover diverse countries such as Cuba, Mexico and others in South and Central America. But in general evidence suggests that the longer immigrants have been resident in the US, the more obese or overweight they become. These findings are not accounted for by socio-economic circumstances, and seem to be clear evidence of cultural 'adaptation'.

Elsewhere, Roshania and colleagues (2008) have looked at age at arrival and its impact on obesity, using a sample of 8500 immigrants to the US. The relationship between obesity and length of residence depended on how old the immigrants were when they moved. Those aged under 20 years on arrival, and who had lived in the US for more than 15 years were almost 11 times more likely to be obese or overweight than those of similar age at arrival but who had only lived there for under 12 months (Table 7.1). This reflects reported dietary change; those arriving at a younger age are more likely to modify their diet, or (perhaps more accurately) to have this modified by exposure to lifestyles at high school. Fennelly (2007) suggested that 39% of a sample of over 6600 immigrants in the

Table 7.1   Adjusted odds ratios of obesity/overweight, by age at arrival in US

Length of residence	Aged < 20 years at arrival	Aged 31-40 years at arrival
Under 1 year	Reference group (1.0)	Reference group (1.0)
1-5 years	3.76	1.19
More than 15 years	10.96	2.31

Source: Roshania et al. (2008: 2673)

Note: Odds ratios are adjusted for sex, education and region of origin

US were consuming more 'junk' food and meat, and less fruit, vegetables, fish and rice, since arriving in the country. Increased sugar and fat intake, and reduced consumption of vegetables and fruit among immigrants has been observed in other studies and represents a negative form of 'acculturation'.

These findings are repeated in Europe. Lindström and Sundquist (2005) examined the impact of country of birth in a Swedish sample (surveyed in 1994) and found that both Arab men and women who had immigrated in or before 1989 had an increased risk of obesity compared with those born in Sweden; they ascribe this to low levels of physical activity.

There is, then, evidence that the 'immigrant advantage' deteriorates over time. Newbold (2005) reports in his study of Canadian immigrants that self-assessed health declines rapidly as little as ten years after immigrants have arrived. His research seeks to understand how the transition from healthy to unhealthy status happens. He suggests that immigrants who are young (20-49 years), physically active, and have a language skill, were less likely than others to become unhealthy, while those lacking a high school education were more likely to show a transition to an unhealthy state. More recent immigrants (those arriving between 1990 and 1994) experienced quite dramatic decline in health status when compared with earlier immigrants and with those born in Canada.

In general, immigrants have better health than native-born counterparts but any health advantages appear to erode over time. The evidence, particularly from the US, suggests that immigrants adopt negative aspects of American culture in relation to patterns of food consumption. There is also evidence of poorer access to health services, possibly caused by a mix of cultural (language) barriers but also structural issues, including discrimination. Set against these issues, of course, are the positives of acquiring new skills that offer access to job opportunities and improved socioeconomic status.

Population mixing

I want in this final section to consider briefly an interesting area of research on migration and health, the focus of which is on internal rather than international migration.

A substantial research literature has emerged during the last 25 years on the impact of in-migration on the risk of disease, in particular, leukaemia. This was prompted in part by the need to understand why there were apparent 'clusters' of childhood leukaemia in the vicinity of nuclear power stations. While some claim that such elevated risk of leukaemia is due to exposure to radiation there are others who suggest that the explanation lies in the high degree of population mixing. According to this hypothesis, relatively stable populations are challenged by being exposed to new infections brought into the area by in-migrants (for example, those working in the nuclear industry). Leukaemia clusters are therefore explained as a rare response to population exposure to (as yet unidentified) viruses.

Leo Kinlen and his colleagues have, in a series of papers, sought to test the hypothesis by looking at areas within the UK that have been subject to high levels of population mixing; for example, new towns, areas to which children were evacuated during wartime, and areas with high proportions of service personnel or migrant construction workers. In an early paper he looked at new towns created after the Second World War that took people from a wide range of locations and compared the incidence of childhood leukaemia with a second set of overspill new towns that took people primarily from London (Kinlen et al. 1990). He found a significantly elevated risk of leukaemia in the first set of towns, suggesting that mixing up people from different places might be a factor in the disease. Research elsewhere confirms these findings; in Ohio, USA, those counties with more than 10% population change between 1990 and 2000 showed elevated rates of childhood leukaemia (Clark et al. 2007), though population turnover is a rather crude way of assessing 'mixing'.

Stiller and his colleagues (2008), in a study of childhood leukaemia in England and Wales, sought to refine the measure of population mixing. They used 1991 Census data to construct a measure of migration diversity; in other words, variety in the set of electoral wards from whence in-migrants of all ages had come during the previous year. Small areas with higher incidence of the disease among children aged 1-4 years took people in from a more diverse set of origins. But, clearly, population mixing (here, diversity of origins) is only a surrogate for the volume and diversity of infections entering a discrete area. In a study of childhood leukaemia incidence in France Rudant and colleagues (2006) look at the joint impact of population mixing, relative isolation, and population density. They argue that there are more likely to be susceptibles in isolated communities, not yet exposed to infections, and that population density represents the propensity for contact (and hence spread of infections) between local residents. They find an increased risk of leukaemia for very young children in isolated areas that have witnessed in-migration but are of moderately low population density.

These studies are suggestive of a relationship between population mobility and the incidence of leukaemia, though much of the evidence is indirect and until there is more direct evidence of an infectious agent the causal link will remain speculative. Such direct evidence will be very difficult to secure, since many infections, especially those in childhood, are likely to remain undiagnosed.

Concluding remarks

Unlike the previous chapter, the focus here has been primarily on voluntary migration, that undertaken to better one's life or that of one's family. It might be motivated by economic factors, taking up new employment for example, or by family circumstances, such as an expanding family or the need to be closer to other family members for social support. Much of this migration, we have seen, is selective of those with better health and this needs accounting for in studies of health inequalities. If relatively healthy people move from 'deprived' neighbourhoods, and therefore leave behind a relatively less healthy population, the gradient of the relationship between ill-health and socio-economic deprivation will steepen.

Those who migrate are, in general, in better health than those left behind or those in the new host population. But we have also seen that those relative health advantages weaken over time, as immigrants adapt their behaviours (particularly their dietary and exercise behaviours) to new norms. And some immigrants find it hard to adapt to new environments, with worsening mental health as a result. The kinetic elite, those moving from one high-powered job to another, can perhaps cope with the transition to a new home overseas, since their employers may provide the means whereby they can adapt better, or return frequently to their former home. Others may not be quite so fortunately positioned in a globalising world, and their relative lack of network capital disadvantages them accordingly.

Part 3: Diffusion

One of the key organising concepts in medical and health geography is, as noted in Chapter 1, that of spatial diffusion; the spread of disease across geographic space. I want to couple consideration of this with ideas, also introduced in Chapter 1, of how the structure of spatial relationships evolves over time; in other words, how improvements in transport have brought places closer together.

Consequently, in the first of two chapters I examine disease spread under conditions of what I call here (following Ulrich Beck) 'first modernity' (see Chapter 1, pp. 3-4 above). This is to suggest that transport technologies were less developed than they have come to be in the late 20th and the 21st centuries. In effect, I am interested in the spatial diffusion of infections overland or via water routes. In the following chapter I look at the spread of diseases that are usually referred to as 'emerging' or 're-emerging'. So the focus there is on diseases that have only been recognised in the last 30 years or so, or on infections that experts had considered of largely historical interest. A focus will also, in part, be on spread that relies on modern air travel; spread under what I refer to as conditions of 'second modernity' or, more simply, a globalising world in which communication is speeded up.

Bacteria and viruses can be spread in four ways (Mangili and Gendreau 2005). The first is *direct* (body to body) contact or *indirect* transmission via the sneezing, coughing or talking of an infected person; the droplets are transmitted over short distances (less than a metre) to a susceptible. Related to this is *airborne transmission* in which the droplets can disperse more widely and remain in suspension for lengthy periods. Third, we speak of *common vehicle transmission* in which infected food or water transmits the infection to many individuals. Last, *vector-borne transmission* is where the disease is spread by insects or small mammals; malaria or dengue fever are examples.

Classic geographic accounts of spatial diffusion make much of the distinction between 'contagious' and 'hierarchical' diffusion. The former suggests that spatial spread is shaped by simple geographic proximity, while the latter proposes that spread is down the urban hierarchy; domestic transport networks that connect major cities serve to structure spread such that places that are close in geographic space get 'leapfrogged'. The distinction has some uses, though the terminology lacks clarity. It is perhaps most useful to think of spatial spread as being constrained by geographic distance under first modernity, while in second modernity the spread is via a series of transport networks that permit rapid spatial diffusion. An alternative terminology might contrast spread in geographic space with diffusion in 'networked' space.

Chapter 8
Disease Spread in First Modernity

Introduction

I consider in this chapter the mobilities of five diseases, in a variety of historical contexts. First, I examine the impact of smallpox on the demographics of native middle and south American Indian populations in the 16th century. Next, I look at the spread of bubonic plague, before turning to cholera, influenza and measles. Clearly, I cannot do more than scratch the surface of disease spread, and the reader must turn to more specialist books and papers for in-depth treatments. My aim is to uncover some of the mechanisms of diffusion, in particular the mobilities of the actors involved, and the ways in which historical transport networks structured such spread. Some of these diseases are still very much with us, but in this chapter my focus will be on the historical context, and I defer to the following chapter a consideration of the impact of more recent strains of influenza.

Smallpox and the conquest of the New World

In seeking to explain the massive reduction in the Amerindian populations in the 15th and 16th centuries many writers have stressed the importance of Spanish domination and barbarity; deaths due to conflict were thought to have wiped out much of the native population. But for authors such as Cook (1998) and others a 'new paradigm points to the unleashing of a series of deadly epidemics as the principal consequences of European expansion' (Cook 1998: 12). Among such epidemics, smallpox was the first to cause devastation and, as Cook has it, 'the worst killer of the Columbian exchange' (Cook 1998: 60).

The disease was first introduced by the Spanish into the Caribbean islands, in late 1518 and early 1519, spreading to the Yucatan Peninsula on the mainland and then north by 1520. The infection reached South America several years later, in 1527, but spread well south 12 months later. The virus could be transmitted by direct bodily contact (including via clothing), or inhalation of airborne particles exhaled by those already infected. Once infected the incubation period was 8-10 days. Since none had experienced the infection before, the entire Amerindian population was at risk, and Cook estimates that 90% of the Amerindian population was killed by imported infections. As the Europeans arrived by ship the coastal areas succumbed first, before spreading inland, either via major river systems or on foot. Later, in the 17th century, new epidemics of smallpox devastated parts of both South and North America, aided by the mobilities generated by the transatlantic slave trade (see Chapter 6). As Cook (1998: 206) puts it succinctly: 'From the Caribbean to coastal Brazil, and northward to New England and New France, no group was spared, although highland peoples fared relatively better than those living along humid tropical coasts'. Clearly, geographical remoteness was something of a protection against viral mobility.

Other deaths in large numbers were due less to smallpox and more to starvation, given the absence of fit people to tend crops and livestock. Further, smallpox was only one of several epidemics of infectious disease transmitted by those from the Old World. Others, also devastating throughout the 16th century, included measles and typhus, influenza, and plague (Cook, 1998). It is to plague, but in a different spatial context, that I now turn.

The spread of bubonic plague

Bubonic plague is a zoonotic disease caused by the bacillus *Yersinia pestis* and transmitted to human populations by the bites of fleas that are infected with the bacillus, the fleas having themselves fed on the blood of wild rodents, particularly rats, that carry the bacillus. Bubonic plague therefore arises directly from the insect bite; primary pneumonic plague arises from exposure to droplets exhaled by other victims or those carrying the bubonic version.

There is plenty of evidence to suggest that plague epidemics occurred well over 2000 years ago. Epidemics in the 6th century coincided 'with Byzantine military operations during emperor Justinian's wars with the Goths and the Persians' (Cliff et al. 2009: 74), suggesting that troop movements played a part in disease spread. The consequences for population decline were devastating, and the disease is thought to have played a significant part in the decline of classical civilisations in the eastern Mediterranean.

Plague is most clearly associated with European mediaeval society and the 'Black Death' is known to generations of schoolchildren. Cliff et al. (2009: 75) posit two possible origins; one, well east of the Caspian Sea, perhaps Mongolia or Tibet; the other, further south in Iraq or Kurdistan. McNeill (1976: 150) asserts that it was the intensification of caravan movements overland, under the auspices of the Mongol empire, that was responsible. 'A communications network comprising post messengers capable of travelling one hundred miles a day for weeks on end, and slower commercial caravans and armies' rendered the Eurasian continent permeable to that empire's reach. Wild rodents of the Asian steppes were infected by the *Yersinia* bacillus. The evidence on spread from Asia across Europe is quite clear. It reached Constantinople in 1347, then south to Egypt and the Levant and westwards through Italy a year later, France and then Britain, where spread was from the south coast in 1349, into the Midlands in 1350 and the north-west of England and Scotland by 1351. The epidemic had run its course by 1352, by which time some 25 million people are thought to have died in Europe. Wonderfully detailed maps of the spatial diffusion are given in Christakos et al. (2007).

The rate of spread was incredibly rapid, perhaps several kilometres each day. The conventional wisdom is that spread was along trade routes. But not all 'nodes' on these trade routes were affected. Milan and Würzburg, for example, were relatively unscathed (Nutton 2008: 8). Moreover, bubonic plague is not transmitted directly from human to human. These sorts of anomalies have led some to question whether *Yersinia* was indeed the causal factor in the Black Death. Scott and Duncan (2004) consider that something akin to the modern-day *Ebola* virus was more probable and agree that spread was due to viral transmission via direct human contact. They suggest that the virus was transmitted 'by travellers, religious pilgrims, and fairgoers travelling along established trade routes…and spread through contact with bodily fluids or inhalation of aerosols produced in sneezing or coughing' (Bossak and Welford 2009: 751). They argue that the summer peaks in mortality were due to the mixing of travellers and traders and that as such population movement subsided in winter months the spatial spread also subsided. Those areas that were not impacted by the virus were exposed to fewer movers, or restricted their entry.

Plague epidemics returned in the late 19th century and spread across the globe, primarily via shipping movements. The burgeoning ports of Canton and Hong Kong were the origins in 1894, and from there plague-infested rats were carried across the oceans in ships, leading to outbreaks in major ports, such as San Francisco, Rio de Janeiro and Sydney. McNeill (1976: 157) suggests that when steamships travelled faster and carried larger rat populations, the oceans suddenly became permeable as never before. As a result, the disease spread to Indian ports in 1896 and from both south China and India diffused to Australia in 1900. From India it had spread to South America by 1899-1903, from China to the west coast of the USA by 1900 and from South America and Africa to Europe in 1899-1900. All this spread was driven by late 19th century innovations in the size and speed of steamships (Cliff et al. 2009: 486). Nutton (2008: 75) suggests that the outbreaks were confined to coastal areas. However, Christakos and colleagues (2007: 709) assert that Nagpur, in central India, a major trade centre, was well connected by the Great India Peninsula Railway to parts of British India and that the railway speeded up the spread of bubonic plague in India. 'Cawnpore (a railway junction in the United Provinces) and Bhagalpur (the administrative and marketing centre in Bihar with railroad connection) were both infected by more severe bubonic plague attacks than the remaining areas in the region' (Christakos et al. 2007: 709-10). Six million persons died as a result in the late 19th century.

In the twentieth century there were much more spatially confined outbreaks, for example in Vietnam in the 1960s (associated with population displacement accompanying the war) and parts of central Africa. Significant localised outbreaks continue to be reported in central Africa in the first two decades of the 21st century. McNeil (1976: 154) contended that there is a reservoir of plague infection in the western US, with infection propagated from one rodent community to another, propagation that is accelerated by human agency. 'Ranchers actually transported sick rodents in trucks, sometimes across hundreds of miles, with the intention of infecting local communities of prairie dogs and reducing their numbers, thus allowing cattle to find more grass'. Clearly, the spread of a zoonotic infection such as this relies on human intervention, as we shall see in the next chapter. The Centers for Disease Control (CDC) continues to report up to 15 cases each year, in northern New Mexico and Arizona.

I introduced in Chapter 1 the notion of quarantine as a form of spatial barrier to impede the mixing of infected people with those uninfected (susceptibles). Cliff and his colleagues (2009: 601-37) have traced in very great detail how these strategies were implemented in the pre-unification Italian states, over four hundred years, in order to control the spread of plague. Northern city states such as Venice and Genoa had major concerns because of their location as key nodes on the maritime trade routes from Asia and the Levant. They set up collaborative networks of communication to inform each other about suspected outbreaks, a system that pre-figures the modern-day cross-national controls 'and the voluntary relinquishment of discretionary powers by fully sovereign states in the matter of public health' (Carlo Cipolla, cited in Cliff et al. 2009: 606). An extensive and dense network of forts and observation posts was set up around the eastern Mediterranean and the Adriatic coasts to prevent the landing of boats except at fixed quarantine stations. This was a form of 'defensive isolation'. Those suspected of carrying the disease were confined at the isolation hospitals ('lazarettos') for the statutory 40 days.

The spread of cholera

Cholera is a disease caused by the bacterium *Vibrio cholerae*. If ingested it can multiply in the digestive system and leads to severe vomiting and diarrhoea, and, if untreated, death. Transmission is not usually person-to-person; predominantly, the infection is transmitted by the ingestion of water or food that is contaminated by faecal matter. The 'mobilities' of cholera – its spatial spread – arise from the movement of people who contaminate water bodies as they travel or migrate from place to place. As the historian David Arnold (1993) put it in his study of 19th century India, cholera was a disease of migration.

The 19th century origin of the disease seems to be the Ganges-Brahmaputra region of North East India (Cliff et al. 2009: 81). The first major outbreak originated here (in the hinterland of Calcutta – now Kolkata) in 1817, the spread beyond aided by British-imposed flows of goods and army personnel (McNeill 1976: 262). Before then the spatial spread was more restricted, assisted by Hindu pilgrimages and festivals that drew to the Ganges delta large numbers who returned home to infect others. After 1817 there was further diffusion inland, carried by British troops to India's northern frontiers. But more dramatic was the spread to China, Indonesia and Japan between 1820 and 1822, aided again by the movement of British troops, but now by ship. A new epidemic emerged in Bengal in 1826 and, again, military movements carried the disease to the Baltic by 1831 and thence to

England, Ireland, and the US. Cliff et al. (2009: 86) map the spread of both the first and second cholera pandemics.

McNeill and others (for example, Zylberman 2006) stress the importance of pilgrimage to Mecca in the spread of cholera in the mid-nineteenth century. 'Each successive pandemic increased in extent and severity, reflecting the expanding reach of the global transport system and increased movements of people, particularly on religious pilgrimages' (Tatem et al. 2007). During the 19th century McNeill claims that pilgrims returning from Mecca to North Africa and South-east Asia invariably exposed others to the disease. Zylberman argues that the pilgrims generated a 'double contagion', one of which was political (the spread of Islam), the other health-related (the spread of cholera). After the middle of the 19th century faster steamships and rail travel helped to accelerate global spread. Zylberman (2006: 25) reminds us that the Suez Canal opened in 1869 and intensified the spread by reducing travel times. Pilgrims returning to Egypt from Mecca on board a ship in the Red Sea were detained in a camp in the Sinai, in appalling circumstances, if there was a suspected cholera case on board. There were gross inequalities in treatment, with wealthier pilgrims in a position to bribe the authorities for earlier release.

In a classic paper the American geographer Gerry Pyle (1969) mapped the spread of cholera in the 19th century US. There were three epidemics: 1832; 1848-9; and 1866. Pyle's interest was in examining the relationship between the nature of diffusion and the changing structure of transportation. In 1832 the spread was in three paths, all via water-based transport. First, the disease spread from the east, via the St Lawrence River and Great Lakes inland to Canada. The other two paths originated in New York City, one spreading inland via the Hudson and Ohio River networks, the other heading south down the Atlantic east coast. The second epidemic was also spread by water transport (with origins again in New York but also New Orleans). But by 1866 the railroad had arrived and spread was based less on geographic distance and more on the connectivity between major cities that the railroad was joining up. Diffusion was down the evolving urban hierarchy, with larger towns, in general, the first to succumb (Figure 8.1). But there were exceptions; for example, the disease reached San Francisco over 12 months later than would be expected because of its population size, probably because the transcontinental railroad had yet to reach the city (Meade and Earickson 2000: 273).

Patterson (1994) undertook a parallel study to Pyle's in 19th century Russia which endured at least six pandemics through to the early years of the twentieth century. Traditional, and evolving, transport systems shaped the course of the epidemics. 'Nineteenth century Russia, with its ... extensive long-distance trade and labor migration patterns, provided excellent conditions for cholera transmission, especially in the summer months' (Patterson 1994: 1171). For example, in 1830 the disease reached Astrakhan on the Caspian Sea, moving rapidly up the Volga River as barges and sailing vessels made their way north. In the next wave of infection (1848) refugees and migrant workers spread the disease as they left the cities either to escape the infection or to return home to work in the fields. In 1853

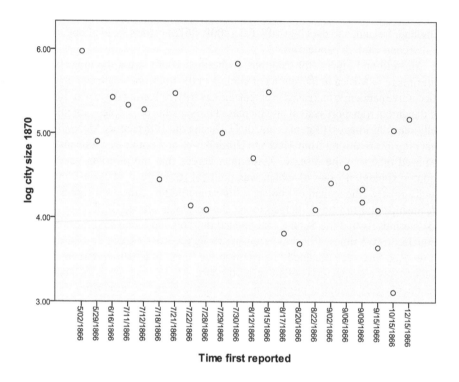

Figure 8.1   Spread of cholera through 1866 urban system in US

Note: Based on data in Pyle (1969): 73.

disease transmission was aided by the emergence of an embryonic rail network as well as by troop movements, rail travel supplementing navigable rivers as a means of facilitating long distance spread. By 1910 the Trans-Siberian railway ensured that cholera could extend its reach all the way to the Pacific, ensuring that this was Russia's first national epidemic (Patterson 1994: 1185). Despite this, disease spread was largely a function of geographical distance, not position on the urban hierarchy as it appeared to be in the latter half of the century in the US.

Cliff and his colleagues (2000) have traced the spread of cholera in the Philippine Islands in the early years of the 20th century, suggesting that spread was affected by the US-Philippines war (1899-1902). The conflict arose as a result of Philippine opposition to US annexation of the islands. Cholera spread through the archipelago (of over 7000 islands) in two waves, one peaking in October 1902, the other in August 1903. In the first wave spread was south by native sailing boats ('bancas') and north by rail from the capital Manila but spread was also to other major centres of population, aided by movements of the American army (Cliff et al. 2000: 282). Cholera diffusion in the second wave seems to have originated independently in three centres of population and to have been more associated with movement linked to post-war reconstruction.

Although accounting for very few deaths in comparison with the major nineteenth century cholera epidemics, the epidemic that broke out in New York City in 1892 says much about the relationship between mobility, class and disease. Markel (1995) offers a richly detailed account of the 'victim blaming' of Russian Jewish immigrants. As is well known this group was one of a wave of European immigrants in the late 19th and early 20th centuries. But this particular group had fled Czarist persecution for the then relative safety of Germany and dozens of ships left Hamburg for New York City. Many of the immigrants had been infected with cholera in very poor living quarters in Hamburg, and cramped living conditions on board did little to halt the onboard spread of disease. As 'the other' the group were stigmatised as 'riff-raff' and 'a positive menace'. 'As the *New York Herald* editorialised, there existed a clear equation of danger: immigrant Russian Jews equalled cholera' (Markel 1995: 426). The response was in part to confine and mix healthy and ill immigrants on the ships themselves, and on isolation islands. It also involved treating different classes of passengers unequally; those in steerage were inspected, disinfected and detained, while cabin-class passengers were examined briefly and allowed to land. The twenty day quarantine period that was deemed appropriate applied only to the poorest passengers, not to cabin passengers, even though they had travelled from the same infected German port. Markel makes the point that the newly arrived immigrant is invariably treated as a scapegoat; his study adds considerable empirical historical weight to this argument.

The spread of influenza

Influenza is a viral disease transmitted from person to person as droplets are exhaled from an infected person ('infective') and inhaled by others ('susceptibles'). The nuclei droplets can remain suspended in air for up to an hour. Some infectives shed more virus than others, and this affects transmission potential, as does the proximity of infectives and susceptibles and the extent to which they are crowded together. Low humidity and low temperature also appear to aid virus survival and transfer; hence the winter epidemics (Cliff et al. 1986).

The epidemic of influenza that spread across the world in 1918-19 is thought to have killed up to 50 million people, very many more than the conflagration that preceded it. As with other diseases, I do not offer a fully rounded account of the pandemic; rather, I again draw on evidence that connects it with the mobilities of various population groups and (in view of subsequent fears of 'swine flu' considered in the next chapter) proximity to animals.

Some claim that the pandemic originated in New York City in 1918 and that the virus was transported to Europe by American troops sent to fight in the final stages of the First World War. Oxford and colleagues (2005) suggest the spread was more likely westwards, with an origin (in 1916-17) in the vast British Army camps that had sprung up in France. During the winter of 1916 there was immense traffic of young soldiers passing through army camps such as that at Etaples in northern France (Oxford et al. 2005: 942). By September 1917 more than a million soldiers had passed through on their way to the front lines, while in the hospitals up to 23,000 wounded were treated at any one point in time, having arrived on one of the ten trains each night from the Somme. The overcrowding provided perfect conditions for the spread of influenza. But Oxford and his colleagues posit that the camp's large piggery, coupled with the purchase of live chickens, geese and ducks from nearby markets (see the telling photographs in Oxford et al. 2005: 943), provided the right conditions for cross species transfer of avian influenza. Demobilisation in the late autumn of 1918 then provided opportunities for further person-to-person spread as soldiers returned by sea and rail to their home countries (Oxford et al. 2005: 943).

The disease is thought to have spread from France to Spain (a neutral country in the First World War) via the return movements of unskilled Spanish (and Portuguese) workers who had been providing a source of cheap replacement labour while young Frenchmen were fighting (Trilla et al. 2008). But other factors aided spread. Traditional holidays at the end of the summer were held all over Spain, and these, along with gatherings for Catholic mass, also provided for the rapid spatial diffusion of the disease.

In an interesting case study of Nigeria Ohadike (1991) examined how disease spread was shaped by transport structures. In late summer 1918 an ocean liner carrying infectives docked in Lagos, Nigeria. Locals were infected and carried the disease inland, reaching Ibadan (on the western rail route) three weeks later. Further ocean vessels arrived at other Nigerian ports, such as Warri, spreading the infection by road to neighbouring towns. 'Once the epidemic had penetrated Nigerian seaports, it made its way into the interior following trade-routes, such as railway lines, motor roads, rivers and caravan routes, progressing "according to the speed of normal transport prevailing on each highway"' (Ohadike 1991: 1395), as a senior public health official reported at the time. Kano, the major city in the north of Nigeria, was infected by late September, with the disease spreading to other towns in the north, such as Maiduguri, Sokoto and Jos. Disease spread was assisted by those seeking to escape the cities; in Port Harcourt about one thousand workers left their jobs and returned home, thus introducing influenza into previously unaffected settlements (Ohadike 1991: 1396). Hogbin (1985) documents similar findings in South Africa. Soldiers demobilised in September 1918 brought back the virus from Europe and ticket records reveal that they boarded trains to stations across the country. Echoing Pyle's research on cholera, she found that the disease spread hierarchically, reaching large inland towns first, before returning to attack those in smaller towns that had previously been bypassed. The response of local authorities was along racial lines, with ticket sales to black Africans restricted while whites were, initially at least, permitted more freedom to travel. Regardless, only the most isolated places escaped infection. Hogbin points out that the relation between the disease and the railway was reciprocal; while the ease of travel increased the speed of disease spread, the resulting infections disrupted the rail service because of the illness or death of so many railway staff.

Quarantine proved largely ineffective in inhibiting disease spread. In West Africa, Liberia banned ships from entering the country's ports in 1918, but the disease entered the country via overland trade routes. In Australia, quarantine was more successful. Vast numbers of Australians, in relation to population size, served in Europe, and returned home on ships in late 1918 and early 1919. But any ship reporting influenza was quarantined in harbour and troops were not allowed to disembark until the infection had run its course. Once on land, travel between states was closely monitored, in some cases by armed guards. Cliff et al. (2000: 195) note that the effect was to restrict death rates in comparison with the USA and elsewhere, though Curson and McCracken (2006) suggest there were around 15,000 deaths and some two million Australians infected.

The 1957 influenza pandemic arose first in southern China (February) – hence it is sometimes called 'Asian flu' – and spread to Hong Kong in April, then across the globe within six months. It 'diffused directly along world communication routes including early "seeding" by air travellers, and indirectly leap-frogging movements with transmission at intermediate points such as European holiday resorts and seaports' (Learmonth 1988: 115). Drawing on Hunter and Young's (1971) geographical analysis, Learmonth points out that ships' crews were key agents of transmission, landing at (then) important ports such as Liverpool, Hull and Middlesbrough in the north of England, from whence the disease spread south. Active cases from India and Pakistan were on board ships that docked in Liverpool and at Tilbury (London) in mid-late June. Britain, being very much a maritime nation in the 1950s, was particularly susceptible to the introduction of influenza by disembarking passengers and ships' crews. Also significant were manufacturing cities inland, with emerging immigrant populations employed in the textile industries. The close proximity of mobile people on commuter trains and on the London Underground also aided transmission as aerosol droplets from infected people were easily inhaled by susceptibles (Hunter and Young 1971).

The spread of measles

Measles is a viral disease, spread through respiratory contact; a susceptible can inhale droplets exhaled by an infective. A highly contagious disease, it has an infectious period of up to 14 days. High rates of vaccination in the global north mean that outbreaks are relatively uncommon, but in the global south, particularly Africa, the disease can be devastating. Historically the disease caused many deaths. A measles outbreak in 1529 in Cuba, introduced by the Spanish, killed two-thirds of the natives who had previously survived smallpox. Mexican populations were similarly affected in the first half of the 16th century, while 1 in 4 of the Fijian population (up to 40,000 people) died from a measles epidemic in 1875 (Haggett 2000: 53-65).

The British geographers Andrew Cliff and Peter Haggett have been at the forefront of attempts to understand the spatial diffusion of measles (see, among many other contributions, Haggett 2000 and Cliff et al. 2009). As they and others have noted, measles shows distinctive wave-like behaviour, with peaks every year in densely populated countries such as the US, every two years in Britain, and perhaps only every 3-4 years in sparsely populated countries such as Iceland (an island 'laboratory' much studied by Haggett's team). A critical population size is needed to sustain the disease; without a sufficiently large population ('threshold' in the epidemiological literature) the disease disappears before being re-introduced by a new infective from outside the region.

As with other diseases my concern here is to illuminate the ways in which movement facilitated disease spread. Looking first at the Fijian epidemic of 1875 it is clear that the virus was introduced by the return to Ovalau Island, Fiji (on board a British ship) of the island chief and his family, who had contracted the disease in Sydney, Australia. The chief entertained many visitors arriving from other Fijian islands to welcome him home; they in turn returned home to infect others, while other British ships carrying measles docked at island ports. In the latter half of the 19th, and early 20th centuries, waves of Indian immigrants to Fiji, working on sugar cane plantations, arrived on ships carrying infectives. Haggett (2000: 62) reports that 1 in 3 ships left Indian ports with measles cases on board. But much depended on whether the ships were under sail, as in the late 19th century, or steam (late 19th and early 20th centuries). On the slower ships, with fewer passengers and longer journey times (3 months), any on-board infection had time to die out; on faster, more crowded, ships (1 month from India to Fiji) the disease could pass from person to person, the infective period ensuring that people landed carrying the disease. Infection by those on board ships also characterized the arrival of measles in Iceland in the early 20th century (Cliff et al. 2009). In particular, the major epidemic of 1916 started with the arrival in Reykjavik of a ship from Norway, carrying a sailor infected with measles. The disease spread across the island.

In a detailed analysis of the growth of international shipping destined for the US Cliff et al. (1998) point to the important role this had in introducing measles. The number of vessels arriving at US ports more than doubled between 1850 (c. 10,000) and 1870 (26,000 a year), falling as the size of ships increased. Again, they point to the important transition from sail to steam, dissolving the relative epidemiological isolation previously enjoyed by the US. Analysis of journey times to the two major ports, New York and San Francisco, suggests that a solitary incubating case of measles leaving some Latin American ports would still be active when arriving in the United States, with the capacity to start an epidemic (Cliff et al. 1998: 50).

The importance of travel by road is stressed by Bharti and colleagues (2010), who examine regional and local transmission of measles in Niger, West Africa. Niger encounters measles epidemics during its dry season, when people have moved from lower density agricultural areas in the rainy season, to higher density urban areas. But added to this seasonal movement is a high degree of 'epidemiological connectivity' to nearby places. Six districts in Niger show higher than expected incidence of measles (1995-2004) and all are closely connected, via the road network, to adjacent Nigeria, which provides a reservoir of infected cases. Although the authors lack detailed data on migration they assert that the six districts are likely to receive significant influxes of people. Thus a core area (Nigeria) is 'spatially coupled' to a periphery into which the disease spreads via the road network.

Concluding remarks

The importance of overland and waterways travel is clear from these examples. Human movement and disease spread were slow relative to the examples I consider in the next chapter. Contact between native populations and European settlers were crucial in spreading infectious disease, and the relative location of aboriginal populations was important. Those that were peripheral and managed to avoid economic (trade) contact were less at risk than others. Diseases such as those considered here, as well as others, spread via inland waterways and, later, via rail routes. Well-established trading routes became the main networks enabling spatial diffusion. But it would be a mistake to imagine that an epidemic of one disease followed another of the same, or different, infection in some kind of linear sequence. The infections often accompanied each other. As Herring and Sattenspiel (2007: 194) indicate with reference to the 1918 influenza pandemic, being exposed to tuberculosis early in life increased the chances of dying from influenza later in life. Diseases interacted with one another, as they continue to do so.

What we witness in the examples considered here is spread in geographic space that is shaped by simply spatial proximity or by emerging transport networks; road; rail, and steam-ship. The diffusion process is speeded up by transport developments; such developments help places 'converge' in time-space (see Chapter 1, pp. 9-10). In the next chapter we shall see how the process of time-space convergence accelerates, to bring places across the globe within just a few hours, rather than days, of each other.

Chapter 9
Disease Spread in Second Modernity: Emerging and Re-emerging Diseases

Introduction

I want to turn my attention now to the diffusion of disease in the latter years of the 20th century and the first part of the 21st. I focus in part on diseases (such as tuberculosis) that have been with us for many years but have re-emerged strongly, in part associated with relatively new infections, such as human immunodeficiency virus (HIV). Since both are, to a large extent, diseases that impact most acutely on the poorest people in society, it is appropriate to place these in the context of global inequalities. Next, I examine diseases that bind animals and humans into new networks, examining the spread of strains of influenza that can cause illness or death among human populations, I also consider the spread of foot and mouth disease, since the mobilities of cattle (and humans, to an extent) are relevant to the discussion.

I devote special attention to severe acute respiratory syndrome (SARS). While this, and the other 'networked diseases' discussed here are of major public health concern, it has to be said that the attention of the public, and of policy makers (academics too), is – compared with the major 'killer' diseases of inequality – rather disproportionate to their global health burden. There is a clear distinction between diseases such as SARS which emerge suddenly but are of short duration and those such as HIV/AIDS and tuberculosis, which are shaped by underlying poverty and inequality. Further, the language used differs according to the disease. Thus the metaphors used to describe the latter, and the accompanying immigrant 'menaces' in some cases, are of 'flood' and 'deluge', with 'swamp' describing the burden placed on hospital services (Coker and Ingram 2006).

After considering some infections that are associated with the movement of goods, in the final section I examine the extent to which infectious diseases might be spread by those seeking to disrupt social, economic and political life in the global north; disease used as a weapon to inflict 'terror' on the public.

All the examples considered here have in common the broad global context in which they are situated. This is one in which the speed of transmission is potentially very fast, such that places which are geographically separated by perhaps thousands of miles find themselves close together in what we might call 'disease space'. But the context is quite different from that considered in the previous chapter, where spread was by road, water, or rail. Here, it is transmission by air travel that merits considerable attention. Second modernity (what some call late or liquid modernity) provides the space-time context. What happens locally is shaped by events far away in geographic space but close in time-space; as noted in Chapter 1, this is a defining feature of globalisation.

Air travel in the early 21st century is characterised by three features: the large volume of passengers moving from place to place; the increased speed of travel over long distances; and the density of networks or inter-connections. There are obvious consequences for disease transmission and, in particular, the ability to detect new outbreaks, since a short incubation period may mean that an infected individual boarding a flight in (say) Canada – and not obviously unwell – reaches the destination (say, India) and only presents with an illness some days after arrival, by which time many others may have been infected. They in turn spread the disease via their contact networks.

Cliff et al. (2009: 26-29) draw on earlier work by Stephen Morse that proposes a set of six factors contributing to the emergence and re-emergence of diseases. These are:

1. Microbial adaptation and change – microbial evolution, emergence of antibiotic resistance
2. Ecological changes – changes in land use, including agriculture and deforestation
3. Human demographics and behaviour – population growth, urbanisation, migration
4. International travel and commerce – the worldwide movement of people and goods
5. Technological change – changes in food production, transport of blood and tissue products
6. Breakdown in public health – poor sanitation and vector control, global conflict and population displacement

It is clear from this simple list that 'mobilities' are implicated in all sets of factors, but most explicitly in 3-6.

However, to this set of characteristics we can add others. In some cases (SARS is a classic example) the nature of the new threat is uncertain and unpredictable. In addition, while transport and technological change matter, it is the blurring of the global and local that matters in many cases. Last, an understanding of (re) emerging infections demands an acknowledgement of the networking of human and non-human elements.

Mobilities of disease in an unequal world

I referred in Chapter 5 to the risks of HIV/AIDS faced by those working in, or participating in, sex tourism. Here, I take a broader perspective. De Carvalho and her colleagues (2010) have reviewed data on HIV infection among international migrants. While there is a danger of over-generalisation, it appears that many, though not all, studies reveal that rates of HIV infection are higher among migrants than for the general population in the destination country. The authors report that two-thirds of HIV cases reported in the UK were most likely acquired (probably through heterosexual sex) in Africa. But while some migrants acquired HIV before leaving, others acquire the infection after migration, or as a result of return visits to high-risk countries. For example, HIV prevalence among Haitians living in Canada were doubled among those Haitians who returned frequently to Haiti, while among Surinamese living in the Netherlands the risk of HIV infection was also associated with travel back to Surinam (de Carvalho et al. 2010: 18).

As Tatem et al. (2007: 300) acknowledge, 'certain groups of mobile and sexually active individuals are important in seeding local epidemics, including immigrants, intravenous drug users, tourists, truck drivers, military troops and seamen'. Gandy (2008) paints a decidedly structuralist view of HIV transmission, suggesting that the structural adjustment programs imposed by the World Bank have had a serious impact on the sexual health of women. 'In a common pattern, truckers, migrant workers, and other men who must travel in order to earn enough to support their families frequent brothels and then infect their wives' (Gandy 2008: 176). Early cases of HIV infection included 'Patient Zero', a Canadian flight attendant whose sexual contacts in several American cities helped diffuse the disease as those sexual partners in turn infected others (Gould 1993). Elsewhere in his polemical book Gould asserts the importance of the airline network in Africa in spreading HIV. But unlike others, he stresses the role of the kinetic elite in the diffusion process; the business travellers; the military officers; politicians; and various 'experts', all part of an international African circuit with access to rapid transport. Taking Abidjan (the capital of Ivory Coast) as an example, sitting 'like a great spider in the middle of a web of direct [airline] connections' (Gould 1993: 84) he refers to it as the 'sexual crossroads of Africa', a node in the airline network that (at least, in the 1980s) acted as a hub through which many passed, being infected by, and infecting, individuals who continued the chain of transmission.

Further evidence of the importance of mobility in spreading HIV comes from a plethora of studies, many focusing either on long-distance travel by truck drivers in the global south (see the brief discussion in Chapter 3 above) or on the seasonal migration of labourers. A study in West Africa (Lagarde et al. 2003) showed that those leaving rural areas for overnight or short-term visits to urban areas adopted more risky sexual health behaviours, and were more likely to be HIV positive, than those who were not mobile. However, as noted by Camlin and her colleagues (2010), much of the literature on migration and HIV risk focuses on mobile men. Their study of migration, gender and HIV risk in KwaZulu-Natal, South Africa, suggests that women, far from being passive recipients of HIV infection from male migrants, participate fully in the migration process and therefore bear a considerable share of the burden. Their study population (of almost 12,000 adults) is highly mobile, with over one-third having moved within the previous two years. Among those who were migrants, 43% of women but 'only' 24% of men, were HIV positive. Female migrants were twice as likely as male non-migrants to be HIV positive. Clearly, such women are deeply embedded into the socio-spatial networks that continue to spread the virus. Working in the informal sector, with less exposure to workplace health promotion schemes and with pressures to offer sex in exchange for material goods and money, puts them and network contacts at risk.

It is, of course, not sufficient simply to study the migrant 'paths'; it is important to ask about the socio-economic context of both the origin and destination, as well as the length of time since migration (see also the discussion in Chapter 7). While migration may disrupt social networks, the extent of such disruption will depend on whether there were supportive social networks and protective social norms at the origin, and whether the place was a site of relative advantage or of poverty. At the destination, migrants might find themselves lonely (and therefore perhaps engaging in risky sexual behaviours) or, alternatively, embedded into strong social networks that might not sanction risk-taking. If moving (or forced to move) to an area where employment prospects were poor new migrants might be faced with the need to engage in transactional (and possibly risky) sex in order to support themselves and their families. Greif and Dodoo (2011) explore some of these ideas among over 2300 female 'slum dwellers' in Nairobi, Kenya. Their results suggest that those who migrate from relatively well-off areas have a 'protective buffer that can attenuate the internalization of negative slum norms and messages, at least initially'. But these effects disappear after living for some time in the slum. Deane and his colleagues (2010) have called for more nuanced consideration of migration, criticising those social epidemiological studies that adopt overly simplistic measures of mobility status. What matters, they argue, is understanding the specific context of, and motivation for, mobility.

Tuberculosis (TB) is a highly contagious bacterial disease that spreads when an infected person coughs droplets into the air and these are inhaled by others. Until the mid 20th century when antibiotics became available the public health response was to confine those infected in TB sanatoria, a form of quarantine that *immobilised* those who would otherwise be mobile and a risk to others, though such sites were also considered places of rest, care and treatment.

Recent data from WHO suggest that the prevalence of TB across the globe is 2 billion, with 1.8 million people dying from the disease in 2008. Incidence of the disease increased during the 1990s (in part associated with the rise of HIV infection and the development of TB that proved resistant to drug therapies) but there is clear variation from country to country. In much of western Europe estimated incidence rates are low and have been falling since 1990; but in parts of sub-Saharan Africa the rates are high and often increasing (Table 9.1). As the table indicates, rates in North America are low. However, there is evidence to suggest that rates of infection in the US are high among immigrant populations; Coker and Ingram (2006: 161) quote evidence that, in 1998, of just over 18,000 cases of TB reported in the US, 41% were in foreign-born people. Nonetheless, the case rate has been falling steadily since the 1990s among the foreign-born in the US (Bernardo 2007). In the UK, 67% of cases in 2002 and 71% in 2005

Table 9.1   Estimated TB incidence (cases per 100,000)

	1990	2000	2007
France	26	16	14
Germany	20	11	6
Spain	56	35	30
UK	12	12	15
Sierra Leone	207	377	574
South Africa	301	576	948
Sudan	174	212	243
Uganda	163	340	330
Zambia	297	602	506
USA	9	6	4
Canada	10	6	5

Source: WHO Global Tuberculosis Database.

were of people born abroad (Gilbert et al. 2009: 647). Disaggregating by ethnicity, Coker and Ingram (2006: 170) note that the incidence rate in the UK among black Africans born abroad was 366 per 100,000, a figure that is clearly little different from those living in Uganda (see Table 9.1). Gilbert et al. (2009) suggest that the increasing incidence in the UK is due largely to the fact that there are relatively high levels of migration from countries with high incidence of TB. Research by the Health Protection Agency (HPA) indicates that in 2010 the number of cases in the UK was the highest for 30 years (9040 reported cases). The HPA suggest that people have either caught the disease before migrating to the UK or have been infected on return trips to their country of birth (www.hpa.org.uk/NewsCentre/Na tionalPressReleases/2010PressReleases/101104TB/).

Evidence also suggests that there is little transmission from immigrant to native-born populations (Craig 2007). Such transmission as does occur is within high-risk clusters of people, such as a migrant community or the homeless. 'The rare exceptions to "within community" transmission often attract media attention and increase public concerns related to TB and foreign-born residents' (MacPherson and Gushulak 2006: 716). Boyle and Norman (2010: 354) note that the incidence of disease is less to do with immigrant status *per se* and more to do with the poor housing and other indicators of socio-economic status; once this is controlled for higher rates among immigrant groups decline in statistical significance. As Susan Craddock (2008) notes, the association between the prevalence of TB and immigrant populations is invariably regarded as a tight one, leading to calls for the 'targeting' of the foreign-born in addressing this as a public health problem. But she points to evidence suggesting that in New York City and San Francisco in the 1990s few new cases in US-born populations were transmitted by immigrants. Further, many immigrants only develop the disease several years after arriving in the US. There is clear evidence of victim-blaming or 'tropical thinking', with the 'tropics' designated as the location of disease and the first world the 'locus of health, biologically threatened when boundaries disappear or fail' (Craddock 2008: 192). There is, she argues, too much focus on *who* is diseased, and not enough on *why*, and too much emphasis on *containment* rather than *eradication* (see also Craig 2007). Controlling TB in countries of high incidence would seem to make more economic and public health sense than worrying about the immigrant 'menace' (MacPherson and Gushulak 2006). Further support for this approach comes from work by Dye and colleagues (2009) which suggests that TB incidence declines more quickly in those countries of the global south that have lower child mortality, good access to sanitation, and score highly on a human development index.

Convery et al. (2006) have contrasted the different 'borders' for TB screening in the UK and Australia. Screening for entry to the UK has, typically, not been undertaken at the point of departure, or offshore, or at the port of entry; rather, at the local destinations within which immigrants have been concentrated. Thus the 'border' (if it can be regarded as such) has been more internal than external. In Australia the screening has been offshore rather than at the point of entry. As Convery et al. (2006: 110) express it, the equivalent (for Australia) of Ellis Island in the US was, historically, Australia House on the Strand of London, where applications for emigration from the UK were processed. More recently, the 'hoops through which to jump' (Convery et al. 2006: 100) are now more numerous for those applying to migrate from other countries (for example, from south-east Asia). Policy in the UK (where the immigrant 'menace' has, over time, shifted from the Irish, to those from the Indian sub-continent, to eastern Europeans and now refugees in general) is currently orientated towards screening in the origin country (presently parts of the Indian sub-continent, some countries in west and east Africa and south-east Asia). As the UK Border Agency puts it: "This programme is part of our 'firm but fair' policy on immigration and will benefit the UK's public health by preventing the entry into the UK of infectious tuberculosis sufferers until they have been successfully treated" (www.ukvisas.gov.uk/en/howtoapply/tbscreening/, accessed 22 August 2010).

Mobilities of viral disease: on cows, birds, pigs – and hybrids

The focus of attention in this section is on diseases that are 'zoonoses'; those with an animal origin. I begin with a discussion of foot and mouth disease (FMD) which caused major social and economic disruption in Britain in 2001, resulting in the culling of animals in over 2000 farms in order to contain the spread, and a loss of some £9 billion to the economy.

Transmission of FMD is from an infected to a susceptible animal, with very few virus particles required to infect another animal. Transmission was, in 2001, aided by the movement of animals to auction marts. One such market, Longtown (in Cumbria, the worst affected county), 'was at the epicentre of a maze of 25,000 animal movements across the UK between February 13th and 16th. By Thursday

March 1 Cumbria's first case was confirmed' (Convery et al. 2008: 27). That case had arisen as a result of a sheep transported from Devon, in the south of England. The government response was to cull (slaughter) susceptible animals both from farms that had been infected and from farms, often adjacent (contiguous with infected farms), that computer model predictions suggested were likely to be infected. The slaughtered animals were then buried or incinerated on pyres that burned for a long time and were highly visible markers of the disease. Subsequent evidence (Convery et al. 2008: 29) suggested that this culling policy over-estimated the risk of local spread and failed to recognise local geographies; Cliff et al. (2009: 322) refer to studies showing that major roads served as barriers to movement in some cases; this was because the cattle bridges crossing motorways were closed. Restrictions on movement, and mass slaughter, proved to be the main policy instruments to deal with the disease. Personal and professional travel was greatly restricted, the public was asked to stay away from the affected rural areas, and footpaths were closed. 'Fears that every tyre-tread and every pair of muddy boots could be harbouring FMD resulted in dramatic alterations in public movement...Through the lens of biosecurity, event-goers of all stripes appeared as potential threats to a delicate national ecosystem' (Johnson 2009: 143). The 2001 outbreak of FMD has been used in science and technology studies (STS) as a prime example of the importance of non-human objects in transmitting disease. Such objects include: other animals; farm buildings and machinery; the distribution of foodstuffs; and the wind. As Adey (2010: 191) puts it, the 'mobilities of the organic and the inorganic, the animal and the human are "coimplicated"'. Convery et al. (2008) offer a detailed description and analysis of the 'emotional geography' of the outbreak, drawing on rich qualitative data (from interviews and diaries) of the 'insiders' – those closest to the disaster.

The first point to make is that, in common with other disasters there are impacts on both individuals and communities; the individual suffers trauma, but there are collective effects on the social body. Thus for the farmer 'to see your life's work lying dead in your yards and fields is something no-one can imagine until you see it for yourself' (cited in Convery et al. 2008: 57). The relationship between a farmer, the farm as 'place', and the livestock is an intimate one and its fracturing was truly traumatic. Understandably, the disposal of the slaughtered animals was devastating for many, including farmers and their families, local residents, and others forced to drive past or see them. The pyres of burning carcasses were hugely distressing visible reminders of what was likened to an 'animal holocaust', where 'witnesses told of the sky being darkened and likened the sight of flames and heavy black smoke to the burning oil wells following the Iraqi invasion of Kuwait and the first Gulf War' (Convery et al. 2008: 43). Although treating FMD as an infection characterising late modernity, the simple but visible and devastating incineration was, in effect, mediaeval technology (Convery et al. 2008: 74). The materials used on the pyres – straw, coal and wood – were common, and took on roles that were quite different from normal farm use. The impact on vets and government officials was also devastating for some; as one of the latter put it: 'I'll never be able to look at a cow or a sheep again without seeing blood pouring out of the hole in its head, maybe I will in time...I walked, walking along the pier one night. I did actually think about jumping in...I felt so bad about myself' (quoted in Convery et al. 2008: 123). Indirect impacts on health and well-being included loss of income; visitor numbers to rural areas dropped sharply, such that those running businesses (hotels, restaurants, pubs, guest houses and shops) catering to tourists and visitors suffered loss of livelihood. In sum, the mobility of the virus, and the subsequent loss of mobility of human populations, greatly affected community health in Cumbria and elsewhere in Britain.

Direct contact with animals – in particular, poultry such as ducks and geese – has been responsible for the emergence of a new kind of influenza (avian influenza, or 'bird flu': H5N1), initially (1997) in China where many towns and cities host large bird markets. The WHO has noted (Hinchcliffe and Bingham 2008) that it is probably transmitted through exposure during the slaughtering of such poultry and preparation for cooking. The intensification of poultry production, and consequent over-crowding of birds, has facilitated rapid disease spread among the birds. Further, the growth in demand for poultry in Southeast Asia has mushroomed in the last 20-30 years; Kimball (2006: 59) reports that exports from Southeast Asia rose from 200,000 tons in the early 1990s to 1.8 million tons only 10 years later. Cases of the disease in humans result from close contact with sick birds. Meade and Emch (2010: 378) point to spread via bird migration routes as well as poultry trade routes, with cases reported in central and eastern Europe.

As of May 2009 over 430 cases had been confirmed by laboratory tests, with 262 deaths, mostly in Vietnam and Indonesia, but with incidence and mortality peaking in 2006 (who.int/csr/disease/avian_influenza/country/cases_table_2009_05_28/en/index.html). The response, following more recent outbreaks in South-East Asia, has been to slaughter large numbers of birds, with severe consequences for the economies of countries such as Vietnam. Such decimation of the poultry flock occurred elsewhere, as Hinchcliffe and Bingham (2008: 223) document for Egypt, where the response was to justify the imposition of more 'orderly' and 'modern' large-scale poultry production as a means of ridding the country of small-scale producers.

Several studies have looked at the outbreak of H1N1 ('swine flu') in 2009, thought to have led to at least 130,000 human cases, of which over 40,000 were in the US (Meade and Emch, 2010: 378). Mortality is very low (less than 1% of diagnosed cases). In a British context the virus is thought to have entered England via a flight from Cancún, Mexico, to Birmingham (Warren et al. 2010: 728). Khan et al. (2009) sought to use airline traffic out of Mexico to examine spread of the disease. There was a strong correlation between the international destinations of travellers leaving Mexico and cases of H1N1 known to have been associated with travel to Mexico.

In their study of the spread of influenza Grais and colleagues (2003) note the substantial increase in passenger air traffic across the globe since the last major flu pandemic in 1968. At that time some 160 million passengers were international travellers each year. By the end of the century this number had increased to 620 million international passengers. According to Airports Council International the total number of passengers passing through 1200 airports worldwide was 4.8 billion in 2007, up from 3.6 billion on 2003; these much larger figures than those cited by Grais et al. include domestic travel as well. Grais and her colleagues construct a table (matrix) of flows between 52 world cities and then 'seed' an imaginary influenza epidemic in Hong Kong. Analysis of the 1968 pandemic (originating in that city) reveals that cities closest to Hong Kong (Manila, Singapore, Jakarta) were infected first; Sydney was forecast as the 48th city to report cases. However, forecasts for 2000 using air traffic data for that year indicates that Sydney is among the first cities to receive cases, along with Melbourne, Perth (Australia) and Wellington (New Zealand). An influenza pandemic would reach cities in the northern hemisphere over 100 days sooner than it was predicted to do in 1968. But there are of course limitations to the mathematical model. For example, no population sub-groups are analysed. Given that the 2009 outbreak of swine flu (H1N1) appeared to be targeting relatively young people, more sophisticated modelling should take demographics into account. New pandemics may well be structured by international air travel, but once arriving in a country it will be regional and local patterns of movement (especially, at local scales, movements of children and journeys to work) that spread the infections.

Although not concerned with specific diseases, Andrew Tatem has sought to model the likely global dispersal of infections via the worldwide airline network (Tatem and Hay 2007, Tatem 2009). His very imaginative analysis has two components. First, data on flight schedules were obtained for over 2500 airports and over 40,000 routes that helped create the total monthly seat capacity of flights from one airport to another. Second, monthly climate data (temperature, precipitation and humidity) were obtained for the airport locations and a measure of climatic similarity constructed between each pair of airports; in other words, airports that might be thousands of kilometres apart could share similar climatic characteristics. Combining the airline and climate data permits Tatem to identify those routes that both carry high levels of traffic *and* link places that are climatically similar (and therefore likely to be potential 'risk routes' for the transfer of viruses or insect vectors). He also predicts possible growth in traffic between routes, suggesting that increased traffic to and from China, India and Russia will provide further opportunities for 'exotic' species to be imported, particularly in June, July and August when air traffic is at its peak. As Tatem suggests, because of the expansion of the global air network and consequent increases in passenger and freight traffic, organisms now have many more opportunities to expand their ecological ranges.

Other research has examined the strategies used at airports to control disease spread as well as representations, by the media, of global travel. Warren and his co-authors (2001) remind us that the Director-General of the WHO, Dr Margaret Chan, suggested that advice to avoid travel to affected countries (such as Mexico) was fruitless. But while such advice was designed to protect the traveller, there were moral and ethical reasons to restrict travel, such restrictions seeking to prevent travellers themselves infecting, unwittingly, those who might not have access to high quality healthcare. As Warren et al. (2010: 734) put it: these 'representations of the "ethical" long-haul traveller, policing themselves and showing consideration to "others", contrasts with long-established narratives in which the Western traveller sought to safeguard their own health against contamination from the "degenerate" environment of the global South'.

SARS

Severe Acute Respiratory Syndrome (SARS), a form of viral pneumonia, emerged as a problem in late 2002 and early 2003 when an unknown virus appeared in Guangdong Province, China. It is believed to have crossed the species barrier from animal (civet 'cat') to human populations. Precisely how such 'cross-over' arises is not fully understood, but factors such as poor sanitation, the mingling of human and animal habitats, keeping animals in cramped conditions, and the widespread use of antimicrobial agents, all are important (Kimball 2006: 99). From mainland China SARS spread to Hong Kong and Hanoi, Vietnam. The index case (a so-called 'super-spreader') was a doctor in Guangzhou Province who travelled to Hong Kong and infected others in a hotel and nearby apartment block (Figure 9.1). Its spread to Canada and Singapore was facilitated by the volume of flights out of Hong Kong, with onboard transmission, on at least five flights, generating 37 cases of SARS (Kimball 2006: 48). The spatial diffusion of SARS seemed therefore to be a function of initial exposure to animals and access to air travel. Introducing exotic animals, which were stressed and shedding virus, into densely populated areas provided an ideal setting to expose animal handlers and the public to that virus. Clearly, provision of better sanitation and clean water, along with less intensive food production, can help mitigate the spread of the infectious agent; but once the infection is in circulation the volume and speed of air travel aids the spread considerably.

According to the World Health Organization SARS infected over 8400 people in 32 countries, and led to 916 deaths (Ng 2008: 73). The majority (over 90%) of cases and deaths were in China, Hong Kong and Taiwan. Estimates of losses to Asian economies range from $18-30 billion. Disruption to travel was considerable, with the volume of air traffic shrinking considerably; Cathay Pacific normally carries 33,000 passengers each day, but that number fell to 4000 in April-May 2003 (Baehr 2008: 139).

In an important collection of essays, Ali and Keil (2008) and their contributors reflect on how SARS has spread through the network of highly interconnected world cities – those linked through flows of people, commodities, and capital. These inter-connections have grown in recent years as places have 'converged' in time-space and international boundaries become more permeable.

Canada's largest city, Toronto, emerged as very vulnerable to SARS (van Wagner 2008), for the following reasons. First, it is a major hub in the international air transport network and the major Canadian gateway city, with some 35,000

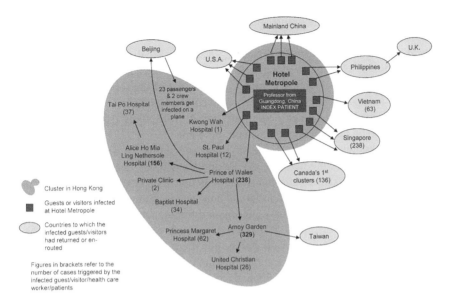

Figure 9.1   Local and global spread of SARS

Source: Reprinted with permission from Ng (2008).

passengers leaving the airport each day. Second, as the archetypal multicultural city it is home to many diasporic communities and a destination for overseas migrants and tourists. Third, the public health system in Toronto was not well prepared for the SARS onslaught, being affected by cost-cutting in the public sector that has led to poor hygiene in hospitals (Keil and Ali 2008a). Budget cuts had led to impacts on physical infrastructure: crowded waiting areas in hospitals, poor infection control, limited isolation rooms and staff shortages. There were further problems in information flow and exchange, with 'work being done in silos' (Keil and Ali 2008a: 60) and outdated computer systems that meant disease surveillance was of poor quality.

In her examination of Hong Kong Mee Kam Ng (2008) confirms some of these findings and adds other dimensions. Hong Kong's fragmented governance structure and budget deficit provided one set of problems, while mainland China was continuing its economic ambitions and lacked a focus on social infrastructure. Ng constructs the major problem for Hong Kong as being a bridge between a socialist country trying to reform and engage with the market, and a globalising world. But the bridge was a poor one, with little evidence of good communication between health and government officials in mainland China and those in Hong Kong.

Ali and Keil (2008a), and some of their contributors, remain unconvinced that a simple network-based approach to understanding the transmission of SARS is wholly satisfactory. For example, van Wagner (2008: 23) suggests that 'there are significant human and non-human aspects of connectivity that are not adequately confronted by our images of network connectivity'. He and others (Schillmeier

2008) demand post-structuralist approaches (such as actor-network theory: ANT). These approaches seek to counter what they see as simple binary divisions between 'local' and 'global' scales; for example, SARS saw local practices translate into a global threat, while those global risks impacted on local practices or social life. ANT also argues against further binary oppositions of the social and the natural. SARS, it is suggested, brought together assemblages of objects; the non-human virus combined with human actors, air traffic, institutions (such as hospitals), media and so on to form a heterogeneous network.

ANT acknowledges the complexity and 'messiness' of disease spread, and the heterogeneity of the network. As Schillmeier (2008: 184) has it: 'the social relevance of the SARS cosmo-politics emerged as a heterogeneous and multiple becoming of, simultaneously, human and non-human, cultural and natural, private and public, local and global, past, present and future, actual and virtual relations, which questioned, disrupted and altered habitual personal and socio-cultural ordering modes'. This may well be so, but there has to be detailed empirical analysis that goes beyond mere contemplation of complexity and messiness.

Hooker (2008) discusses SARS in the context of other health scares, including those that share the same characteristics of producing major fears about potential catastrophes while, at the same time, generating relatively low mortality. As she observes, the disruptions are to economies (trade) and societies (movement of people) but not greatly to human health. The scare arises from 'the rapid movement of peoples and organisms...[and]...agricultural and industrial practices that constantly cross boundaries between species' (Hooker 2008: 129). With specific reference to Toronto, Keil and Ali (2008b) agree with this, suggesting its impact is not as a 'killer' but 'as a destroyer of the tenuous multicultural fabric of Toronto' (Keil and Ali, 2008b: 154). The risks are amplified socially by the network of relations among individuals and places, particularly global cities. But, as Hooker points out, some networks proved beneficial, as when the connectedness of the international scientific community (itself a network) facilitated knowledge transfer about the virus itself. Further, the experience of dealing with SARS has led to improved planning for other potential pandemics (for example, swine flu).

As Baehr (2008) observes, the WHO 'trumped' the sovereignty of individual states by intervening actively in policies to inhibit the spread of SARS. WHO issued advice in April 2003 against unnecessary travel to Toronto; a form of quarantine. The city became 'exotic plaguetown' (Strange 2006), no longer a technologically advanced world city, and it took considerable resource to re-brand the city after the danger had passed. The risk became highly visible with the wearing of masks. This became something of a ritual and an obligation: 'failing to don one was met with righteous indignation, a clear sign of ritual violation' (Baehr 2008: 150). The very visibility of the masks and the extent to which their visibility increased in newspaper and television reports, raised the level of the threat and displaced from the public consciousness the much greater burden of disease and death faced by the world's poor. Toronto in the global north got more publicity than sub-Saharan Africa tends to get as part of the global south.

Mobilities of malaria

Malaria is a disease transmitted by a 'vector'; various species of the *Anopheles* mosquito, which, in its bite, introduces the *Plasmodium* parasite into the bloodstream. Each year, there are more than 250 million cases, with well over one million deaths, particularly of young children in sub-Saharan Africa, where incidence is very high (Meade and Emch 2010: 117). Malaria is commonly associated with poverty; while mosquitoes do not discriminate between humans on the basis of their economic capital, prevention, control and treatment (for example, access to bed-nets and to drug therapies) is unequally distributed.

There is a huge literature on malaria epidemiology and, most recently, the impact of climate change on disease prevalence. As with other diseases, I restrict attention to those aspects that are associated specifically with human movement. I should also add that while attention focuses on contemporary aspects, I could readily have discussed aspects of malaria mobility in the previous chapter, since human movement (for example, of soldiers returning to the US after the second World War, and after the Vietnam War: see Meade and Emch 2010: 121) has long played a part in its spread.

Over 50 years ago the geographer Mansell Prothero noted the links between human movement and malaria incidence (see Gatrell and Elliott 2009: 161-2 for a brief description of his work). These links are as important as ever. For example, Osorio and her colleagues (2004) showed that, among those living in the town of Quibdo, Colombia, residents who had travelled, within the previous 8-14 days, to an area in which malaria was endemic, were almost 30 times more likely to present with malaria symptoms than those who had not travelled. It is not simply the case that movement into high-endemic areas leads to infection; local transmission is enhanced when those infected return home and transmit the parasite to other mosquitoes when they are bitten. These mosquitoes in turn bite uninfected individuals.

Mosquitoes can be inadvertently transported by the aircraft; on arrival any insect bite can transmit the parasite to people in or close to the airport. Since 1969 about 30 cases of 'airport malaria' have been reported in France (Queyriaux et al. 2009). Surveys in India reveal high numbers of insects at all airports and seaports (Sharma et al. 2005), despite the fact that the International Health Regulations (IHR) require that airplanes arriving from areas affected by insect-borne diseases (such as malaria and dengue fever) are systematically disinfected. 'Disinsection' seems to be effective, though Tatem and colleagues (2006) note that the number of countries implementing this is shrinking.

Budd and her colleagues (2009) have traced measures deployed to limit the threat to public health from the expansion of international air travel in the twentieth century. Western countries produced interventions that 'framed certain destinations as being host to an array of "exotic" or "tropical" diseases that represented a threat to health and economic development' (Budd et al. 2009: 427). The chief aim was to maintain bio-security. Interestingly, the threat was understood over 70 years ago, one doctor in 1938 commenting on the danger of yellow fever being spread by passengers incubating the disease or by infected mosquitoes on board the aircraft. These fears were not misplaced; the same doctor noted that half the aircraft arriving in Kenya in the 1930s harboured insects, despite eradication measures. At the same time, others worried that measures to control insect vector movement served to delay flights and were a hindrance to the movements of people and goods. But controls such as 'disinsection' remain in place for some international flights between particular pairs of places.

Tatem, Rogers and Hay (2006) use the same methodology as outlined earlier (p. 141) to estimate the risk of malaria due to air travel. That is to say, the more similar are pairs of airports in terms of climate, and the higher the volume of airline traffic, the more likely is the transmission of *Anopheles* from one airport to another. There are a number of high risk routes in July, August and September; for example, Abidjan (Ivory Coast) to Paris; Accra (Ghana) to Amsterdam; and Entebbe (Uganda) to Brussels. All of these European destinations have previously reported local transmission of malaria. The predominance of African airports in the list of high-risk routes reflects the coincidence of the malaria transmission season and the European summer. In more recent work Tatem and Smith (2010) have examined migration between pairs of countries rather than airports, and have identified clusters of countries which send migrants from areas of high malaria incidence to those of lower incidence. For example, Mali and Burkina Faso are net exporters of migrants and are areas of high malaria intensity that form a migration 'cluster' by virtue of sending migrants to neighbouring countries (such as Senegal and Mauritania) that have lower rates of malaria. Other countries, such as Ethiopia and Myanmar (in South East Asia) are relatively isolated in terms of population flows (at least, insofar as these are reflected in official data) and therefore perhaps less at risk of the parasite being transmitted across national boundaries. Some researchers have begun to use mobile phone data to estimate human mobilities and Tatem and colleagues (2009) have exploited these ideas (together with data on likely exposure in different parts of Tanzania) in assessing the likely importation of malaria parasites from the African mainland to Zanzibar.

As noted by Tatem, Hay and Rogers (2006) the movement of large container ships has also been responsible for introducing new species of mosquito, including those responsible for both malaria and dengue fever. Dengue fever is another vector-borne disease and while it causes far fewer deaths (perhaps c. 20,000 deaths world-wide a year) its distribution too has been associated with human movement. Eggs and larvae of the mosquitoes are carried in pools of water lying in tyres being transported on the container ships. To explore this further Tatem and his colleagues have adopted methods similar to those described above, incorporating data on shipping routes to explore the possible spread of two *Anopheles* species. Of the top ten shipping routes that present the most risk in terms of traffic volume and climatic similarity, seven of the destination ports are those where *Anopheles albopictus* has been detected. For example, Genoa, Italy, has reported the mosquito's presence, and while another port (Fraser, Canada) has not, the climatic similarity to Japanese ports that send large numbers of ships to Canada suggests it may be at risk. It seems likely that air travel was responsible for introducing the same species to Hawaii.

In linking malaria (and other mosquito-borne diseases such as dengue fever) to human movement the recent focus has tended to be on large-scale patterns of movement and broad spatial scales; for example, air travel across the globe. Others have stressed the more local-scale, fine-grained mobilities. In particular, Stoddard and his colleagues (2009) have drawn on ideas of time-geography, of the kind portrayed in Figure 1.2, to suggest that the risk of malaria is a function of differential exposure to species of mosquito in different environments. For example, during the day people are not at risk of being bitten by the largely nocturnal *Anopheles gambiae* (responsible for malaria, and mostly confined to rural settings) while *Anopheles aegypti* (responsible for dengue fever) tends to be more active during the day (and more confined to urban areas). Thus there are certain local environments which, coupled with local mobilities, contribute disproportionately to the transmission of the parasite and hence the disease. Clearly, there are different mobilities at work; the mobility of the mosquito and the mobility of human agents. Linking these to non-human actors (such as the distribution of water pools, the availability of bed-nets and so on) produces an actor-network whose structure requires sophisticated empirical work to unravel.

Mobilities and trade-related infections

I take the term 'trade-related infections' from Kimball's (2006) important book, which examines in detail how infections can spread rapidly in an era characterised by the fast movement of goods and people round the globe. Kimball argues (2006: 3) that a trade-related infection is characterised by three components. First, there is the continuing expansion of production of foodstuffs to meet global demand, expansion that increases the risk of cross-contamination of infections. Second, allied to this is the distribution of such foodstuffs via a network of trade links that shift goods (and thereby, potentially, infections), from points of production to points of consumption. The third component is the impact that the detection of such infections has on the economies of those countries from whence they are deemed to have arisen; countries in the developed north can weather these shocks to the system much better than resource-poor countries of the south.

The pressure to deliver economies of scale has led to the growth of large food production enterprises, squeezing smaller farms out of the marketplace. Kimball (2006: 24) notes that the number of farms in the US declined from 6.3 million in 1929 to 2.2 million in 1998. A consequence is the huge size of cattle herds and the potential for cross-contamination with (for example) *E coli* O157:H7. Numbers of reported infections have risen enormously in recent years. *E coli* infections are not restricted to beef products but can arise from fruit and vegetable products contaminated by infected water supplies.

Along with *E coli*, another example of a trade-related food-borne infection is *Salmonella*. This is traditionally associated with eggs, poultry, raw meat and milk but in recent years has been spread via nuts, fruit and vegetables, probably because of water contamination or transfer from work surfaces or improperly cleaned utensils. A major outbreak in the US in 1994 infected a quarter of a million people and was due to the consumption of ice-cream produced in Minnesota and distributed across the US. The spread was most probably due to transfer in tankers that had previously carried unpasteurised eggs. Other examples of *Salmonella* infection relate to the increased consumption (and therefore trade) of seed sprouts (of radishes, alfalfa and cress), ironically as a result of consumer demand for health foods. The seeds are contaminated by direct contact with animal faeces or are grown in areas close to pastures that are faecally contaminated. Kimball also reports diarrheal symptoms resulting from infection by the parasite *Cyclospora*, linked to import of (water-)contaminated raspberries from Guatemala. This kind of outbreak invites some public health officials to call for better surveillance and regulation – 'the basic radar which allows us to understand when we are under attack by microbiologic missiles' (quotation by Michael Osterholm, Minnesota State Epidemiologist, in King 2008: 206). But it is too easy to fall into the trap of blaming those in the global south when there is plenty of evidence of poor management in the food chain in the north (witness the many farm-related outbreaks of *E coli* O157 in the UK and elsewhere).

The third component in Kimball's argument concerns the severe consequences on local economies from restrictions placed on travel and trade. If the World Health Organisation or national governments advise against travel to areas affected by outbreaks of infectious disease, or trade is restricted, the financial impacts can be severe. Guatemala lost millions of dollars in earnings when the US Food and Drug Administration (FDA) banned imports of fresh raspberries from that country in 1998 (Kimball 2006: 31).

Mobilities and the weapons of disease

The use of biological agents to exert dominance over a particular population has attracted considerable attention in recent years, especially as the threat from terrorist groups has grown. New mobilities are being created that involve movements of terrorist cells across borders, and potential movements of materials needed to wage biological warfare that is far removed from the classic disputes between two or more states. Of course, the use of such agents is hardly new. In the fourteenth century the bodies of people infected with bubonic plague were used as catapult weapons, while the British used smallpox-infected blankets to subdue Native Americans in the eighteenth century (Kimball 2006: 87; Gatrell and Elliott 2009: 35-7).

Two sets of events within the last 20 years have brought 'bioterrorism' to the fore. The first was the release of sarin gas (a deadly nerve agent) by members of the Aum Shinrikyo cult in the Tokyo subway system in March 1995. This killed 12 commuters and seriously injured 54 more. But Aum's public campaign of terror had begun a year earlier when sarin gas was released in the city of Matsumoto, northwest of Tokyo. A neighbourhood was targeted that was the home of judges hearing a case against the cult. A light breeze pushed the aerosol cloud of sarin into a courtyard, killing seven people. At the cult's headquarters other chemical weapons and biological warfare agents were found, including anthrax and *Ebola* cultures (Olson 1999).

The second event was the distribution, in September 2001, of anthrax-infected letters mailed from Trenton, New Jersey to US Senators in Washington and to news media. Five people died and 17 others were infected. The sender of the material has never been confirmed but is thought to have been a government bio-defence scientist who committed suicide after learning of a likely prosecution. There have also been accidental, rather than deliberate, releases of bio-materials. For example, there was a release of anthrax spores from a microbiology and virology laboratory in Sverdlovsk, Russia, in 1979; this killed at least 79 people (Kimball, 2006: 88).

Western governments are also concerned about stockpiled viruses falling into 'rogue' hands. Smallpox is considered a major possible biological weapon, and the break-up of the Soviet Union – which had stored the virus – has for some years worried public health specialists. Routine vaccination against smallpox was discontinued 40 years ago and so only a small proportion of the population would have any immunity if that virus was introduced via a terrorist attack. Like anthrax, it would be highly lethal and easily transmissible by air (Kortepeter and Parker 1999). It is ironic that diseases (such as smallpox, anthrax, and plague) associated with first modernity (Chapter 8) should be the focus of renewed attention in a world of global risk. The lack of medical insurance among poor Americans – and other under-insured populations – would mean delays in seeking health care if any such infections were to arise in the community. This could, in turn, lead to more rapid spread of such infections, not least because of possibly more densely populated communities that enhance the speed of an epidemic.

It is also important to note that the threat, or perceived risk, of such releases is as much of a public health issue as actual events. The anthrax attacks in the north-east US caused panic among the population and widespread disruption to postal services and government business. Residents stockpiled antibiotics that, presumably, remain unused in medicine cabinets. Unscrupulous individuals can take advantage of lay peoples' worries by hoax calls to the media. But while governments have to take any threat seriously, other public health issues (smoking and obesity, and their consequences for human health, for example) dwarf bioterrorist threats in terms of their burden. While the probability of an event is very low its impact will be extremely high. But contrast this with water-borne infections in resource-poor countries, where both the probability of infection and the impacts are extremely high. We need to put into perspective the recent concerns with bio- and agro-terrorism. As Gandy (2008: 184) has noted, 'this Western preoccupation with security is largely irrelevant to the daily threats endured by the poor majority, and especially women, throughout much of the global South'.

'Agroterrorism', or the deliberate contamination of foodstuffs, must also be acknowledged as a mobile threat. A former senior US government official noted upon resignation that 'for the life of me, I cannot understand why the terrorists have not attacked our food supply because it is so easy to do' (quoted in Kimball 2006: 94). Such an attack could be focused on causing direct harm to populations – by poisoning foodstuffs or water supply systems – or by causing irreparable harm to ecosystems. As Kimball (2006: 95) observes, a very small proportion of foodstuffs entering the US gets inspected, and presumably much the same applies at the borders of other countries that might be the target of terrorist groups.

I outlined in Chapter 1 some of the new methods (such as GOARN and GPHIN) for monitoring possible disease outbreaks. These do not rely on case finding among national governments; rather, they use the internet as a form of timely 'syndromic surveillance'. Moreover, data may be collected and analysed that is not directly related to medical assessment; for example, unusual purchases of facial tissues, over-the-counter medications for coughs and colds, high rates of absenteeism from work or school and so on might all be signifiers of a disease outbreak (Weir and Mykhalovskiy 2006: 254). They might help as an early warning system for terrorist-related attacks that use bio-weapons.

Concluding remarks

Many of the concepts considered in Chapter 1 need to be put to work in an understanding of disease spread in the contemporary world. At local scales ideas of time geography and activity spaces are required to understand the spread of tropical diseases in rural areas, or between rural and urban areas. The ways in which transport technologies evolve to bring places closer together (time-space convergence) affect rates of spread, particularly in a global context. Yet there is differential risk and exposure depending on context and the nature of the infection. Some of the diseases considered here are shaped by the distribution of power and resources and their incidence increases as such power and resource access diminishes. Others, particularly respiratory infections such as influenza are, in a global context, shaped in other ways by access to 'network capital'. Frequent flyers (the kinetic elite) may be more likely to be exposed to infections circulating at hotels and airports, and can play crucial roles in seeding new epidemics, depending on the extent to which they come into contact with other groups. Yet despite the importance of global mobility networks in second modernity, more local networks involving mundane mobilities continue to be important and cannot be neglected. Any member of the kinetic elite infected while on a business trip can readily transmit the infection to a family member who can in turn help spread the infection in the local community,

There is a network of actors to study when exploring contemporary diffusion patterns. Ali (2008) suggests that the global outbreak of SARS 'can be conceptualized as the emergent outcome involving the convergence of at least three specific types of flows: viruses, people and information'. Braun (2008: 263) reminds us that public health exists within a framework of 'extra-corporeal systems – flows of air, water, sewage, germs, contagion, familial influences, moral climates, and the like'. He goes on to suggest that the focus of public health policy 'has never been the body in relation only to itself, but *bodies in motion*, in relation to other bodies, to food, and to animals' (my italics). Cities have become 'biosocial', no longer separating us from nature or from rural hinterlands but environments in which animals have become enfolded with human populations. New approaches to understanding spatial diffusion are required that bring together the different mobilities – of vectors, viruses, people, and information.

Finally, it bears repeating that while the disruptions due to some of the disease spread considered in this chapter have been immense and there has been serious loss of life, the burden of disease (and mortality) pales into insignificance compared with that from HIV/AIDS, tuberculosis and infectious tropical disease.

Part 4: Communication and Care

In the final part of the book I turn attention first to the mobility of information and how it is related to care and well-being, and, in a second chapter, to the mobility of health carers and health care.

In Chapter 10 I focus on communication – the mobilities of information. Initially I am concerned with immobility; the extent to which we are sedentary rather than active, and how this affects health. Next, I consider the health impacts of the mobile phone, before seeing how social networking affects health and well-being. Last, I examine how the internet provides the means for online information and support. There is a growing interest, among lay people and those with particular health conditions and illnesses, in creating and maintaining networked communities of care. All these modes help form network capital, capital that can be exploited for health gain. While at times they can engender risk they provide the means to overcome space-time separation in physical space and to form new spaces of virtual care and well-being.

In the final substantive chapter I focus initially on two forms of mobility, both of which are expressions of globalisation. First, I consider the migration of health professionals and, second, I look at the mobilities of those travelling abroad to seek healthcare. Both of these mobilities involve international travel. In the first case movement is of those who produce (deliver) healthcare while in the second the mobilities are on the consumer side. Last, I consider the ways in which health care is both provided, and consumed, remotely. There is clearly an overlap with the previous chapter, since information can be transmitted or communicated that does, of course, in itself provide a form of care. But I pay particular attention to the burgeoning topic of telehealthcare (and its subset telemedicine), which offers care 'at a distance' that may save time and money; whether it does or not, and whether it improves health and well-being, requires careful and critical analysis.

Chapter 10
Mobilities of Information

Introduction

A question of general interest is the extent to which new information and communication technologies (ICTs) modify, or are modifying, human mobility. Does adoption of the internet, mobile phones, social networking sites and other virtual communications media reduce the need to travel? All these technologies have enjoyed considerable market penetration in recent years.

As Stradling and Anable (2008) observe, we might expect the advent of domestic online shopping, business video-conferencing, and social networking all to reduce the need to travel. However, this is not necessarily the case. ICTs might actually stimulate the demand for travel. For example, setting up an online dialogue between firms might subsequently require face-to-face meetings, while those working more from home might substitute leisure travel for the time they would otherwise have spent commuting. Stradling and Anable (2008: 191) suggest that 'when the broader and longer-term effects are studied, on balance ICT generates *more* communication, including new travel' (my italics).

There are considerable benefits to mental health resulting from access to radio communications. For older people, or those with visual or mobility impairments, the radio can act as an essential 'lifeline'. People who have been held hostage for long periods of time (the ultimate immobile) report that the radio has kept them in touch with the outside world and at times reassured them they are not forgotten. The BBC World Service has been mentioned specifically in that regard. In a very real sense both conventional communications technologies such as this, as well as new technologies, provide a means, and an experience, of 'mobility' for those who may be, either temporarily or more permanently, immobile.

Here I pay attention to the impacts on health and well-being that result from forms of *communication* or information exchange. I examine the material objects or devices used for such interactions as well as the interactions themselves, particularly those of an electronic form. To what extent do the things that flow – the forms of information exchange – as well as the material infrastructure that makes these mobilities possible, affect human health?

Couch potatoes and mouse potatoes

I take the sub-heading from descriptions by the journalist McCellan (cited in Valentine and Holloway 2002: 313) which suggest that there is over-exposure to television (on the 'couch') and to computer use (the 'mouse'). What is the evidence with respect to both forms of media?

The economist Richard Layard, in his popularist reflections on *Happiness* (Layard 2005) paints a rather grim picture concerning the impact of television. Echoing Robert Putnam, he asserts that television is destructive of community life and family and social relationships, and that since engagement with it can only be passive it reduces the scope for physical activity. For him the evidence that violence in television contributes to violence in real life is persuasive; for example, reported suicides or those included in television dramas generate suicides in the community. In addition, he considers that television influences happiness by virtue of comparison effects; since social dramas tend (he claims) to portray wealthy people viewers over-estimate the affluence of others, thus lessening their happiness. Last, 'television creates discontent, by bombarding us with images of body shapes and riches we do not have' (Layard 2005: 90).

In terms of impact on physical health, the fact that television viewing is sedentary in nature invites us to assess whether excessive exposure is associated with lack of physical activity and, perhaps, levels of obesity. There will always be debate about what an 'appropriate' level of exposure might be. Data suggest that the average time spent watching television is 28 hours a week in the US and 22 hours in Europe (de Wit et al. 2010). Children's food preferences are still targeted via television, especially advertisements. Kelly et al. (2008) have studied this in Australia, examining over 700 hours of broadcasting and the advertisements carried by commercial broadcasters for food, using premium offers (competitions) and promotional characters such as those in cartoons. Of the 20,000 advertisements shown, a quarter were for food, and they predominated at peak viewing times. Persuasive marketing techniques such as these promote brand recognition and product preferences. Advertisements for fast food are rather more common than those for fruit and vegetables! Beyond this the evidence is patchy and of doubtful value. Consider two examples cited by Ray and Jat (2010). In the first, a study purports to show that watching more than two hours of television a day (coupled with lack of parental control over viewing) is associated with an increased risk of early sexual initiation. Second, and equally controversially, the frequency of viewing violent films during childhood is possibly associated with violence and delinquency in adolescence. These are serious social issues, but whether the associations are genuinely causal is debatable and it would seem that carefully designed studies (with adjustment for other factors) are sorely needed.

A recent longitudinal study conducted in Quebec, Canada is one such example (Pagani et al. 2010). Parents of children aged 29 months were asked about weekly exposure to television. At 10 years of age the same children were assessed for a range of health behaviours and academic achievement. Results suggested that, after adjustment for confounders, every additional hour of TV viewing led to a 6% reduction in mathematics scores, 13% reduction in time spent on physical activities, and 10% increases in consumption of snacks and soft drinks. For these authors, lack of mobility in pre-school settings predisposes such children to unhealthy adolescence. The concern is that time spent watching TV is time that could be spent on healthier activities, including play and developing friendships.

Turning to the impacts of television viewing on mental health, some research shows an association between sedentary behaviour (including television viewing) and anxiety and depression. A recent study of British children (Page et al. 2010) suggested that higher levels of TV viewing (and computer use: see below) were related to psychological difficulties. However, as noted by de Wit and her colleagues (2010) there are various possible explanations; mental ill-health could be due to lack of physical activity, or to social isolation, or to TV exposure, or the latter association could be reversed (i.e. those with mental disorders watch more television). Their own study of 2300 Dutch adults confirmed a strong association between those suffering from panic attacks and agoraphobia, and television viewing, but did not provide evidence for causal association. It seems entirely conceivable that being confined to one's home as an agoraphobic is almost inevitably likely to lead to increased viewing; it is less convincing that exposure to TV induces agoraphobia!

The same considerations apply to the use of computers. Evidence suggests that respondents with major depressive disorders spend more leisure time than a control group using computers (de Wit et al. 2010). This contrasts with evidence from other studies which suggests an inverse association between use of the internet and depression; as noted later, if the internet is used for online chat it might serve to reduce the incidence of depression.

In recent years there has been considerable interest shown in using the television monitor to connect interactive computer games, particularly those 'exergames' (notably, Nintendo® WiiFit) that help improve fitness, balance, and rehabilitation after illness. The WiiFit extends the use of the Wii video game console (which does not itself improve energy expenditure or physical activity) by combining a balance board (rather like bathroom scales) with the Wii games console; the pressure sensors in the board detect shifts in balance. Among older adults, where falls (and hence fractures) can be a serious problem, WiiFit has been shown in a small-scale Scottish study to improve balance (Williams et al. 2010). All participants enjoyed the exercise and gained confidence as a result. Studies are required to see if this kind of intervention improves fitness and reduces levels of obesity that are of contemporary public health concern.

Mobilities and the mobile (phone)

My primary focus here is on the mobile phone, a technology whose availability has grown exponentially in the last 20 years. But we should not forget the importance of the landline in delivering social support. Consider just one example. In the previous chapter I described the devastating impact of FMD on farmers and others in the UK during the 2001 epidemic. Hagar (2009) has commented specifically on the information needs of farmers, showing how – given the severe restrictions on human movement – farmers relied on the landline both for information and emotional and social support. Simple 'talk' helped, and the telephone was preferred to email as it had immediacy and a human voice. The one-to-one communication provided 'psychological first aid' (as Hagar puts it), while special help-lines helped disseminate information and provide additional support.

Lefebvre (2009) suggests that, in 2009, over 3.3 billion people world-wide have a mobile phone, and that these are therefore almost ubiquitous as a communications medium; the number of texts (short message service – SMS) in the US grew from some 81 billion in 2005 to 363 billion just three years later. Kwan (2007: 435-6) reminds us that AT&T had estimated, in the early 1980s, that there would be about 1 million mobile phone users in the US by the year 2000; in fact, there were 100 million! She also reveals data on the per capita adoption of mobile phones in 2004, suggesting that in parts of Europe (Luxemburg, Sweden, Italy) there are more than 100 phones per 100 persons, while in Canada and the US the ratios are 45 per 100 and 61 per 100 respectively. No doubt these figures are well out of date already.

The mobilities and connections provided by the mobile phone have been outlined in the recent popular exposition by Christakis and Fowler (2009). They describe a study by González et al. (2008) that analysed sample data from 100,000 anonymous mobile phone users, which allowed the authors to plot the distances between users' locations at consecutive calls (over 16 million such distances were analysed). While the data set is novel – as well as vast – the results are not so surprising; 'people devote most of their time to a few locations, although spending their remaining time in 5 to 50 places, visited with diminished regularity' (González et al. 2008: 781). It is at home and in the workplace where most of these calls get made. Consequently, while the authors are able to describe the statistical structure of human movement (at least, in one un-named part of the global north) the notion that this research illuminates our '*understanding* individual human mobility patterns' (their words, my emphasis) seems exaggerated.

Mobile phones (and other forms of interpersonal communication technology) help to maintain and develop social networks and social support. They connect people on the move rather than at fixed places. As a socio-technical resource that maintains and nurtures relationships they provide network capital. The very transportability of the medium means that calls or texts can be sent, in principle, anytime and anywhere (though not, legally, while driving); in particular, they can be used during otherwise 'dead' travel time. Drawing on detailed interviews and diaries of a small sample of 32 respondents in London, Rettie (2008) suggests that phones help develop more supportive social networks, whether among immediate family members or 'weaker' ties. For one of her respondents the phone was a 'lifeline', claiming that after he has sent his daughter a text: " 'Sent' and I know she's got it, you know, then maybe a couple of minutes later 'ping' I've got a message. *And I find that it's very warming. It's love you know*" (Rettie 2008: 298, my italics). Clearly, such interaction can contribute to a sense of mental well-being, potentially on behalf of both sender and recipient.

Rettie (2008) contrasts mobile phone calls and text messaging, showing how both provide social support, but in different ways. Phone calls are viewed as more supportive than texts, as they are more like face-to-face interaction. As another of her respondents, Anne, said "if I am feeling, um, kind of a bit needy or vulnerable, then text isn't enough. *Then I do need to have a proper dose of somebody*" (Rettie 2008: 299, my italics). There are clearly some situations that demand conversations rather than the sometimes 'blunt' instrument of a text message. However, some people send 'emotional texts' as a simple vehicle for expressing a 'thinking of you' sentiment, without the need for a lengthy call. Intimate partners may find texting (or email) an invaluable means of maintaining close contact, and in the contemporary workplace this informal yet frequent contact may be easier to undertake surreptitiously than the (possibly observed or monitored) telephone call. Those in the early stages of a relationship can find that texting gives more control over relationship-building, since the partner can perhaps dictate the pace of development. Of course, texting or mobile phone calls can be relationship-damaging when intimate messages or texts are discovered by an existing partner.

Urry's research confirms some of these findings. One of his respondents reports that access to a mobile phone is 'just like having a constant network between all of you'. Arrangements (to meet, for example) can be made almost any*where* and any*time*; conventional clock-time can, to an extent, be replaced by 'the fluid time of mobile communications' (Urry 2007: 173). Ling (2008) argues that mobile phones help to maintain the 'strong tie' relationships that may be originally generated through face-to-face meetings, while social media and social networking sites are used for broader or 'weak-tie' relationships. Use of the technology appears to be socially differentiated, with black and Hispanic populations significantly more likely than white people in the US to use SMS.

What are the advantages and disadvantages of such potentially ubiquitous contact? Among the former we can include the usefulness of a mobile phone during emergencies or problem situations, as when a car breaks down in an unfamiliar or remote environment, or when the last bus or train home is missed and parental 'rescue' is sought. Much useful work can be undertaken on the move, using the phone as a communications device. At the extreme, the mobile phone almost becomes part of the body, with people reporting feeling 'lost' without it. Indeed, one of Urry's respondents says that when he lost his phone 'it was the worst week of my life. I didn't have a clue what I was doing or anything' (Urry 2007: 176).

On the downside, for some people the expectation of being constantly available, or potentially interrupted, may be stress-inducing. Flexible lives, the blurring of the boundaries between workplace and home, and the convenience of interacting on the move may be attractive to many (and Kwan 2007 paints a very positive picture) but there are drawbacks. For Kwan (2007: 440) the 'workplace for mobile professionals...may be the office, the home, the hotel room, the car, or the airplane'. Yet such professionals may feel they are almost under surveillance (Peters 2006: 167, with a nod to Foucault, refers to the 'electronic panopticon') with the 'office' able (or expecting) to reach them anywhere, and perhaps any time. Reduced 'real' social interaction can be isolating. The home environment can be tainted with work-related anxiety (Stradling and Anable 2008: 192). The phone can be intrusive, particularly for those in meetings or at public events, such as the cinema or theatre where, despite exhortations, phones will sometimes ring, thereby disturbing others. Trains in Britain, on long-distance routes, have quiet carriages which are supposed to free other travellers from the chatter of mobile phone conversations; few such conversations will be of interest (except, perhaps, prurient!) to others. And while it is 'good to talk' (as a famous telephone advertisement once suggested) it may be healthier to talk face to face rather than risk the misunderstandings that can result without the visual clues or cues otherwise provided by physical proximity.

Having looked at mobile communications and the opportunities that arise in their use, what role might they play in caring for relatives and friends? Caring involves regular and frequent contact with those who are unwell, disabled, or confined to their home or other place of care. In some cases this contact may involve short distances, but in others it may involve long trips. However, as Urry (2007: 227) has it, '[I]ntimacy and caring can take place at-a-distance, through letters, packets, photographs, emails, money transactions, telephone calls, as well as intermittent visits'. This does, of course, pre-suppose that the person being cared for has access to some of the technologies whose use is implied – such as broadband access to a computer. Older adults may lack such network capital and may indeed prefer a visit in real space as opposed to one in virtual space. One of Urry's respondents indicates that texts and emails cannot wholly substitute for visits: 'I couldn't really stay friends with somebody if I am just messaging them and never seeing them. I would have to see them now and again in the flesh and do things' (cited in Urry 2007: 228).

There have been numerous reports in recent years concerning the possible health risks due to the use of mobile (cell) phones. The suggestion has been that exposure to low-energy (non-ionising) radiation may cause neurological damage (in particular, brain cancers) among heavy users of such phones. Several recent studies suggest that the risks may be exaggerated. A major international study (Lahkola et al. 2008) involved taking detailed histories from 1209 people with meningioma (a cancer of the brain), and 3299 controls. The aim was to assess whether regular mobile phone use (defined as at least once a week, for at least six months), duration of call, and cumulative hours of use, were associated with increased risk. In fact, results suggested a significantly *lower* risk of meningioma among phone users. This is confirmed by a case-control study undertaken by an international collaboration (Interphone Study Group 2010). This took data from 13 western countries, comprising just over 2700 cases with brain tumours and 2400 matched controls, comparing the two groups in terms of mobile phone use. The odds of a tumour were reduced for meningioma and glioma, though there was some evidence of elevated risk among those with highest levels of exposure. As with all retrospective case-control studies there are concerns about the abilities of respondents to recall accurately their levels of exposure. Kan and his colleagues (2008) pooled a series of nine case-control studies that comprised over 5200 cases of all brain cancers and 12,000 controls. As with the previous studies, the risk seemed less in phone users, though for studies that looked at longer-term phone use (more than 10 years) there seemed to be a slightly elevated risk of tumour development. Further compelling evidence to suggest there is no association between brain cancer incidence and mobile phone usage comes from an analysis of time series data in the US. The number of users of mobile phones has risen sharply since the mid-1990s, but the age-adjusted incidence rate of brain cancers has remained stable (Inskip et al. 2010). Even though the rate among women aged 20-29 years has risen significantly, detailed analysis suggests the increases are in the frontal lobe and not those parts of the brain that are more exposed to radiofrequency radiation. Finally, since much mobile phone use now revolves around hand-held texting and less direct exposure to the head, this is further suggestive that any risks of mobile phone usage are negligible.

Concerns have also been expressed about exposure to radiofrequency radiation resulting from proximity to mobile phone base stations ('masts'). Again, such concerns seem to be unfounded. In a major British study Elliott and his colleagues (2010) looked at the exposure of pregnant women to such masts and assessed this against the risk of the child subsequently developing brain cancer (and leukaemia). They took detailed geographic data on addresses at birth and compared the exposure (modelled power output of the base stations) of both cases with child cancer and matched controls (healthy children). There was no association between risk of cancer and exposure to base stations during pregnancy.

Social networking and mobility in cyberspace

Social networking spaces permit individuals to present and articulate themselves, establishing and maintaining connections (Farmer et al. 2009). Over the last 10 years the number of social networking sites (such as MySpace, LinkdIn, Twitter, and – especially – Facebook) has grown, and the volume of interactions therein has proliferated massively. Farmer and colleagues suggest that 25 million people in the UK are presently members of one or more such sites; the most popular (Facebook) now has over 600 million active users across the world, with 250,000 new registrations each day. Pujazon-Zazik and Park (2010) note that, even four years ago, 55% of adolescents in the US who used the internet had a profile on a social networking site, more than double the proportion of adult users. Almost three-quarters use social networking sites to make plans with friends, half use them to form new friendships, but over 90% of them use sites to stay in touch with friends they see often.

Such communication technologies are of enormous value. The mobilities of, and access to, information they offer can help build sets of skills and network capital that improve life chances and therefore health and well-being. Yet one of the problems with access to such sites is that, far from helping to reduce social isolation, they may enhance it. Some may become so addicted to online communication that they lose any skills they may have had, or any interest, in face to face communication. As Parr (2008: 153) has it, new 'ghetto geographies' of online communality might exist for people with mental health problems.

The technologies evolve rapidly and research reported by authors even 2-3 years ago is based on cyber-environments that are now quite out of date. Nonetheless, some of the questionable behaviours are likely to be much the same. A good example of how rapidly research dates is the finding in Valentine and Holloway (2002) that access to a computer in British homes of their sample is between 55 and 73%. In 2008, the figure overall is 72% but in the 10% of households with the highest incomes 98% owned a home computer and 96% had an Internet connection. This compares with 33% of households in the lowest income group who owned a home computer and 26% who had an Internet connection (www. statistics.gov.uk/cci/nugget.asp?id=86). Valentine and Holloway (2002) portray a rather positive view of cyberspace for children and adolescents. While they note that cyberspace is a contemporary site of anxiety the narratives they produce from interviews of 11-16 year olds in Britain do not reveal concerns about well-being. Their own findings counter popular fears about safety and suggest that ICTs are means of developing sociality that adds to everyday 'off-line' social networks. Fears of social withdrawal (and therefore poor mental health) and inactivity (and therefore poor physical health) do not figure significantly in their account.

Interest in what has become known as 'cyber-bullying' has grown in the last 10 years. Cyber-bullying can take many forms but in essence is an extension of 'traditional' (verbal or non-verbal) bullying, although using electronic forms of contact, including social networking sites. For example, unpleasant emails can be sent (perhaps to an individual, possibly to a set of individuals). Such 'hate mail' might include words or phrases that are sexist, racist or disparaging of sexual or other identity. Mobile phones can be used to send text or video that is designed to humiliate and abuse the victim. In recent years the phenomenon of 'happy slapping' has emerged, designed to share video evidence of physical attacks. The proliferation of social networking sites means that profiles can be created to intimidate or defame a person or persons. More seriously, adults can adopt the person of a child or adolescent in order to engage in online 'grooming'. Last, interactive gaming allows players to chat online with anyone they are matched with in a multi-player game. Cyber-bullies can then abuse other players and use threats, spread rumours, and 'lock' victims out of games. All these forms share the following characteristics: anonymity and the difficulties of detection; the prospect of a very large audience as the target becomes exposed not merely to a handful but a web-ful of spectators; the ubiquity of the media used for dissemination; and the difficulties of erasure.

Substantial attention has been given to the risks encountered by children in their journeys through cyberspace. What evidence, as opposed to anecdotal reports, exists to justify parental and others' concerns? Although almost inevitably out of-date, and depending on definitions, Shariff (2008: 44-5) quotes some cross-country comparisons. In the US 75-80% of 12-14 year olds report cyber-bullying; 65% of Indian students claim to have been bullied using mobile phones, 42% of girls aged 12-15 in Australia have experienced cyber-bullying, and an astonishing 84% of Canadian teachers report they have been so bullied. In contrast, Smith and his colleagues (2008) report survey findings among a British sample of 11-16 year olds that about 22% of respondents had ever been cyber-bullied. They also find evidence that girls are more likely to be victims than boys and that bullies were as likely to be girls as boys.

Chisholm (2006) gives a helpful overview of the risks in cyberspace, suggesting that cyber-bullying against girls and adolescent females has repercussions for their mental health and well-being. She suggests that poor policing of the Internet means that these forms of encounters in cyberspace are not so different from those in the lawless 'wild west' of nineteenth century America. Teenagers (and adults) can 'flex' their identities online and present themselves in ways they would not off-line. Cyberspace provides an environment in which they can become less inhibited, disclosing information about themselves that falls into the wrong hands. Girls can enter into what Chisholm calls a 'relational style of aggression', in which rumours are spread, threats made to withdraw attention or affection, and individuals are excluded – behaviours that have long existed in the real spaces of the classroom and playground but are now sometimes played out online. Research on such ostracism has shown that simply being ignored and excluded is sufficient to lead to depression and a lowering of self-esteem (Chisholm 2006: 80). For Juvonen and Gross (2008) cyberspace extends the school environment as a domain for bullying. Their online survey of over 1000 youths in the US (aged 12-17 years) suggested that 75% of the sample had been bullied at school and 66% online; equally, 33% had been threatened at school and 27% online. A statistical model that seeks to predict the experience of cyber-bullying found that being repeatedly bullied at school led to a seven-fold increase in risk of being bullied online.

Ybarra and Mitchell (2008) report results from the Growing Up with Media Survey, a national online survey in the US of almost 1600 young people aged 10-15 years. The survey seeks data on: first, unwanted sexual solicitation (requests to discuss sexual matters or provide personal sexual information) and, second, harassment (rude comments or the spreading of malicious rumours). Fifteen per cent of the respondents reported content under the first heading, and one-third under the second. However, the proportions reported on social networking sites were much lower: 4% and 9% respectively. Internet messaging and chat rooms seemed to be where the problems lay (a view supported by Juvonen and Gross 2008) and the authors conclude that social networking sites are not, in the main, targeted for inappropriate behaviours. There is evidence that young people do not inform their parents about negative online experiences for fear that they might restrict access to sites, and one has to ask if the low reported prevalence of bullying on social networking cites is due to an unwillingness to face the risk of such restricted access (Juvonen and Gross 2008).

What are some of the risks to health that arise from cyber-bullying? To some extent they will mirror those that are a consequence of 'traditional' bullying, though the latter often includes physical attack whereas its cyber-counterpart will be verbal and written. Regardless of the environment in which it occurs, or the technologies used to effect it, 'mental anguish from the social exclusion caused by physical and psychological bullying is sufficient to destroy the confidence of any adult, let alone a child, on whom it can have lifelong effects' (Shariff 2008: 25). Both victims and bullies fall prey to serious mental health problems, including anxiety and depression, and low self-esteem. Shariff cites studies indicating that the health effects are worse for people who are both perpetrator and victim. Among marginalised groups (considered in Chapter 6), such as the children of refugees, the consequences can be enhanced because of an unwillingness to complain. Most distressingly, victims can be so traumatised that suicide is considered the only 'solution' (as the moving dedication in Shariff's book testifies). Dealing with bullying is not easy. Dealing with cyber-bullying will be at least as hard. In part, as Shariff points out (2008: 29) this is because adults imagine it can be controlled and policed, whereas the very nature of cyberspace is that it is largely unregulated and fluid.

As a further illustration of the under-regulation of cyberspace, consider again the subject of sex trafficking discussed in Chapter 6. Hodge (2008) draws attention to the uses of technologies that permit the real-time transmission of information and events to any location that can access the technology. He suggests that one of the first uses of video-conferencing was the live transmission of sexual abuse of young women. Specifically, he refers to a live internet 'show' in Hawaii, aimed at Japanese audiences, where consumers could purchase requests for specific sexual acts. Here, a particular form of what one might call a 'cyber-kinetic elite' derives pleasure from exercising power and control over those who have little agency.

Online support

I have already referred to social networking but my focus here is on the use of these and other technologies specifically for social support; support that people give each other in order to improve their health and well-being. Virtual interactions may complement, rather than substitute for, face-to-face interaction. As Wellman (2001: cited in Urry 2007: 168) notes: 'many community ties are complex dances of face-to-face encounters, scheduled get-togethers, dyadic telephone calls, emails to one person or several, and broader online discussions among those sharing interests'. Urry suggests that the dichotomy between face-to-face and virtual, mobile and immobile, even presence/absence, is being broken down as new technologies become part of our life-worlds.

Lefebvre (2009: 490) argues that the constantly connected consumer is a reality for public health. To what extent is this so? He argues that a benefit is the many-many nature of social networking; messages are not transmitted to small groups but to large audiences, 'a world in which they talk back to us, and just as importantly, with each other' (Lefebvre 2009: 491). The costs of communication and interaction are relatively low and transmission of information is rapid and confers anonymity, at least in principle. For people who are physically disabled, or agoraphobic, the interaction from the privacy and comfort of a home environment is welcome.

Social networking sites dedicated specifically to providing online support have sprung up in recent years. Perhaps the most well-known is 'PatientsLikeMe', which allows users to share their health profiles and search (by age, gender, symptoms, and so on) for those with similar conditions (www.patientslikeme.com/). As of January 2011 there appear to be over 10,000 registered users, with communities of interest covering neurological disease in particular, but also chronic fatigue syndrome and HIV.

Farmer and his colleagues (2009) have considered the uses of social networking sites (Facebook in particular) in relation to medicine and healthcare. They identified over 750 different user groups, of which the most common were patient and support groups. Over 60,000 individuals were associated with groups dealing with cancer and heart disease, though less common diseases (such as inflammatory bowel disease) were represented more than might be expected on the basis of their prevalence. For younger patients with diseases such as this, social networking sites help people compare experiences and treatments, as well as the possible side effects of therapies, in an environment that can be supportive and readily accessed (Farmer et al. 2009: 458). Facebook is also increasingly used by the scientific community, and a major publisher (Elsevier) has an application in Facebook that allows researchers to search for relevant peer-reviewed medical literature.

Several recent studies support the assertion that online support communities are valuable for those people living with chronic conditions. Idriss and colleagues (2009) suggest that virtual communities offer both a valuable educational resource and a source of social and psychological support for people living with the chronic skin condition psoriasis. Half of the 260 patients they recruited from five psoriasis support groups reported that their quality of life had improved since joining the group(s) and 40% indicated that the severity of the condition had improved. As a counter to this, Rogers and colleagues (2009) provide evidence that, for psychological therapy, young adults much prefer this to be face to face rather than over the internet. They recruited 328 respondents from Facebook and undertook an online survey that revealed 80% preferred to disclose symptoms of anxiety and depression directly to a therapist rather than via the internet.

Hester Parr (2008) has been at the forefront of assessing (both theoretically and empirically) the benefits of the internet for creating online or virtual communities that provide support for people with mental health problems. To what extent does the internet help create both a relational social space and the 'emotional proximities' that might benefit people with a range of mental health issues? Parr's studies suggest there are very clear benefits from having discussion forums, chat rooms and the like which can help people overcome feelings of alienation and isolation. Sharing information online 'potentially assists users in forms of self-management involving the choosing of medication, shopping around for care and alternative therapies and accessing various activist networks that perform different versions of citizenships' (Parr 2008: 141). Clearly, network capital is being created and reproduced.

In her empirical work Parr conducted an internet-based survey, via four UK-based mental health online forums. This generated data from 80 respondents, mostly young women and mostly white. The evidence on developing effective communities of support is compelling. As one respondent puts it: 'People are so nice and non-judgmental, they are knowledgeable and willing to help and they made me feel a part of a group after being on the outside for so long' (Parr 2008: 144). Others speak of 'an extended family' and the bonds of trust that develop. Self-esteem is enhanced, experiences, knowledge and strategies are shared, and a sense of belonging is created, such that users no longer feel they carry their burden alone. Moreover, for some the gains they realise online – whether of knowledge or self-expression – can transfer into their offline social worlds: 'Sometimes I think that if it wasn't for the Internet I wouldn't have even developed the social skills that I have' (Parr 2008: 151). For many, the interactions within online forums extend to a wish to engage more actively in debates (about policies, therapies, and so on). Consequently, some seek to campaign for changes in practice, or the law, or to raise awareness of issues of stigmatisation.

It would be a mistake to imagine that these forms of interaction are uniformly positive. Text-based interactions cannot incorporate the visual and other cues that people pick up in 'offline' communications, while (as noted earlier) there are risks in exposing oneself to unwelcome attention. Further, continual online presence may make it even more difficult to sustain relationships offline; connectivity may be restricted to virtual worlds.

Concluding remarks

The internet serves to propagate and sustain vast numbers of online communities. But one should not imagine that the internet merely substitutes for face-to-face interaction. Interactions over cyberspace can occasionally lead to interactions in physical space – some of which, especially those involving children, can be at best inappropriate and at worse very dangerous. However, interactions of a 'positive' sort can result from cyberspace exchanges. As Urry (2007: 164) has it, 'intermittent co-presence is important even within virtual spaces', and meetings can reinforce emotional bonds that may have emerged in cyberspace. For professionals used to exchanging information via email, face-to-face meetings provide opportunities for networking that is imperfectly realised in virtual interactions. The latter are often essential in establishing trust. Urry concludes that meetings in cyberspace will, in general, supplement face to face meetings.

The virtual world allows individuals to escape the social and bodily constraints of the real world in order to create imaginary identities. The use of ICTs becomes embedded into their lives and allows them the freedom to create new sets of friends who are geographically remote. This access to network capital can be positive for mental health and supports people who might need help and reassurance from those they may never meet in person. Equally, the continuing growth of mobile communications – both calls and texting – is liberating and beneficial for many, permitting friends and relatives to keep in touch and, perhaps, ensure that the person they are calling is well.

Chapter 11
Mobilities of Carers and Care

Introduction

The internationalisation of labour – in particular, the increased migration of skilled workers – is one component of globalisation. Given this, I want to explore first the mobility of those delivering care, focusing on the movements from country to country of health professionals – doctors and nurses. I then examine the topic of health 'tourism'; travel abroad to seek health care that may be unavailable, too expensive, or proscribed in the country of residence.

In the previous chapter I looked at the extent to which members of communities that are created online can provide support to each other. This leads me here to consider how health professionals, rather than lay people, can offer care in virtual settings; can the internet be exploited in novel ways to improve patient care and, perhaps, reap savings for healthcare systems? In a section on 'remote care' (care at-a-distance, if you will) I consider the broad area of tele-healthcare and its (medical) subset, telemedicine, together with m-health, the use of mobile devices to assess and improve health status. A large set of applications is considered, along with a critique of the role they currently play, and may play in the future.

International mobility of health professionals

There are enormous global disparities in the provision of healthcare resources, including health professionals (doctors, nurses, and others): see Gatrell and Elliott (2009). Naicker et al. (2009) cite some revealing statistics: African countries have, on average, 2.3 healthcare professionals for every 1000 persons, while North America has 24.8 per 1000. Even these figures mask huge variations between countries, and within countries where the contrast between urban and sparsely populated rural areas can be vast. Tellingly, just over 1% of the health professionals across the globe care for those who experience one-quarter of the global burden of disease. An important question is whether these disparities are exacerbated by the mobility of healthcare workers.

There is an emerging body of evidence on the movement of doctors, nurses, and other health professionals, from country to country. Of particular interest is the possible impact on the economic and social infrastructure of less developed countries in the global south from losing (existing or potential) skilled health workers to other countries. Kingma (2007) suggests we should be concerned about this; those countries struggling to meet Millennium Development Goals are those with the most acute shortages of health professionals and the severest challenges of responding to health needs.

The international movement of health professionals is not a recent phenomenon. During the 1950s concerns were expressed about the so-called 'brain drain' of British medical graduates seeking employment in countries such as the US, Canada and Australia. But from the mid-1960s through to 1980 acute shortages of medical staff in developed countries led to substantial growth in the number of doctors trained overseas. By the early 1980s about one-third of all doctors in Canada, Australia and New Zealand had trained in other countries, and this proportion was about 25% and 20% in Britain and the US respectively (Wright et al. 2008). The migration tended either to be of graduate doctors from one developed country to another, or of physicians trained in developing countries and then emigrating to practice in an advanced economy. WHO statistics revealed that 90% of migrating physicians were destined for the global north, where there have continued to be shortages of health professionals (Wright et al. 2008).

An assumption was that much of this migration would be temporary; physicians were likely to return home following the acquisition of new skills in countries with better-resourced health-care systems. The reality was different. The 'pull' factors of higher salaries, better working conditions, good career prospects, as well as the setting down of family roots (Hooper 2008) meant that such migrants tended to stay put. Equally, the 'push' factors (low standards of living, poor working facilities, and so on) served to encourage health professionals to seek work abroad. Witt (2009) suggests that the push factors have been more significant than the pull ones.

The literature on 'brain drain' has debated whether it is attributable to the aggregation of many individual decisions to leave, or, rather, to wider structural forces, including the deliberate 'poaching' of qualified staff by unscrupulous health services in the global north. Ethical issues are raised in both cases. Why should governments deny qualified citizens the right to seek advancement in more resource-rich countries? Conversely, why should governments, or recruitment agencies, in the latter, denude the healthcare systems in resource-poor countries of their talent? And why should the tax-payer in a resource-poor country help to train a doctor who then seeks employment overseas? (Hooper 2009 would have such emigrants repay the costs of their education before leaving for overseas). These ethical and public policy debates have come to the fore more recently, as countries in the global north have sought to increase medical staffing as demand has grown. Wright and colleagues (2008) suggest that such issues are especially acute in South Africa, where the local demand for healthcare is high because of the AIDS pandemic; here, one-half of the domestically-trained physicians are working abroad. One response of the government is to seek 'backfill' by recruiting from nearby African states, thereby producing a 'medical carousel' (as Eastwood et al. 2005, put it) in which other countries are deprived of well-qualified human capital.

Clemens and Pettersson (2008) draw attention to the considerable definitional problems in researching the international movements of health professionals. In considering, as they do, the movements of 'African health professionals', they ask whether such professionals are those resident in an African country, born in that country, trained in that country, or holding citizenship of that country. Their own analyses consider country of birth and, in constructing a comprehensive data-set, they look at the entire continent, at both doctors (physicians) and nurses, and at nine 'developed' countries as destinations. The focus is on those who had moved sufficiently permanently to be recorded in the most recent Census of the destination country.

Their results reveal wide variations in the proportions of African physicians and nurses residing and working abroad in 2000. In Egypt and Libya fewer than 10% of physicians who trained there work abroad, while in countries such as Mozambique and Angola (former Portuguese colonies) the figure is over 70%. Clemens and Pettersson relate the variations to economic and political instability. Those countries (such as Liberia, Sierra Leone and Rwanda) losing high proportions of health professionals were those that had suffered from civil war in the 1990s, while other countries (Kenya, Tanzania and Zimbabwe) had suffered economic decline. The very poorest countries that have weak medical schools have low emigration rates, while countries with relatively strong economies (South Africa, Nigeria) do better at retaining doctors and nurses.

Brown and Connell (2004) have examined the flows of skilled health professionals from three South Pacific islands – Fiji, Samoa, and Tonga – to Sydney (Australia) and Auckland (New Zealand). They undertook a survey of doctors and nurses both in the island countries and the destinations, the 251 respondents including current migrants, return migrants, and non-migrants. Quantitative data from the survey allow the authors to model the likelihood of a move, or intention to move, in terms of personal characteristics and material circumstances, family circumstances, and country of birth. About two-thirds of nurses and half of the doctors surveyed indicated that the higher income-earning opportunities in the wealthier countries were the primary motivation for a move. Ownership of a house or a business reduced the probability of moving, while there were differences among the three countries, with Tongans more likely to move than Fijians or Samoans. Migrating health professionals were also more likely to have close relatives in the destination countries and to have trained there. A lack of career and promotion opportunities, and relatively poor access to facilities and training in the islands were also factors inducing a move. Thus there are both 'push' and 'pull' factors involved in the migration decisions. The research also revealed the importance of health professionals transferring money back to relatives in their country of origin in order to provide financial support. 'Pull' factors were also at work in a survey of 139 nursing students in Uganda (Nguyen et al. 2008), where 70% expressed a wish to work outside the country, preferably in either the UK or the USA, for financial reasons. Only those who came from rural backgrounds were more likely to want to remain in Uganda.

Brown and Connell (2004) stress that return migration is relatively common and Kingma (2007) refers to brain 'circulation' rather than brain drain. Many skilled health professionals return after perhaps several years away, having acquired additional skills and with resources to invest in property, thereby providing some security for the individual, as well as tax income to the state. Consequently, while there are problems resulting from the loss of skilled staff, there is evidence of benefit if such staff return after a period abroad, and government encouragement of such return migration is to be welcomed as a policy initiative.

There is a sense in which nursing can be considered the archetypal mobile profession (Kingma 2007), and therefore considerable attention has been paid to the international movement of nurses, with some research focusing on particular countries of origin. Kingma (2007) gives a snapshot of the proportions of foreign-educated nurses working abroad. In countries such as the US, Canada, Australia, and the UK the proportion from overseas is between 5 and 10%, while in New Zealand it is over 20%. In Ireland in 2005, 84% of nurses recruited were foreign-educated, most arriving from outside the EU. To some extent, migration of nurses since the 1980s has been a consequence of the structural adjustment policies imposed on some countries by the World Bank and the IMF. These policies required reductions in public expenditure. Kingma (2007: 1286) gives the example of Cameroon, where employment restrictions in the public sector led to a suspension of nurse training and a de-motivated healthcare workforce that triggered a search for jobs overseas. Those left behind encounter increased workloads and poor morale. But while economic reasons have always dictated nurses' search for work in the global north, those arriving in the UK from the old Commonwealth countries (Canada, Australia, New Zealand) did so in part as 'adventurer' or 'backpacker' nurses, where the opportunity to travel (not necessarily to remain for extended periods) was a motivating factor.

There is something of an ebb and flow to those trained nurses and midwives coming from overseas to the UK and being registered to practice (Figure 11.1). The intake from India has risen dramatically since 2000, though has dropped recently; the same is true of Nigeria, though with lower absolute numbers. Of note is the rapid growth in numbers coming from the Philippines since 2000, though this flow has tailed off markedly in recent years. In part, these reductions reflect the introduction of a code of conduct (as well as bilateral agreements between the UK and other countries) to prevent NHS organisations from actively recruiting in countries that can ill-afford to lose trained health professionals. But these restrictions applied only to the NHS; migrants continued to enter the UK to work in the private sector, and some were subsequently able to transfer into the NHS (Witt 2009).

Brush and Sochalski (2007) have examined the case of the Philippines in some detail. Over the years, the Philippines has implemented policies of training nurses specifically for 'export' to the US, Gulf states, and Europe. Financially, working in these countries is extremely attractive; the average annual wage for a nurse in the Philippines is just over $2000 (much lower in rural areas), compared with up to $48,000 abroad. Clearly, very substantial increases in wages would be required to entice nurses to return, even allowing for differences in cost of living. And while some of the wages get remitted home (Kingma 2007: 1292, suggests a quarter of the income of many Filipino nurses gets remitted), there is an accompanying cost

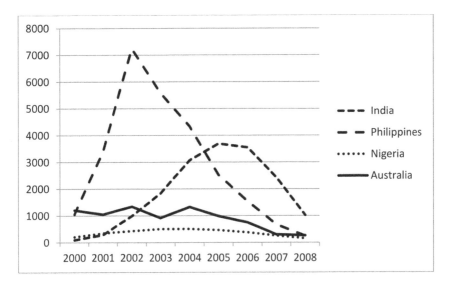

Figure 11.1 Numbers of new nurse and midwife registrations in the UK

Note: Based on data from UK Nursing and Midwifery Council, Annual Registers.

to public health if local needs are unmet. Witt (2009) asserts that the out-migration of nurses from the Philippines has created a domestic shortage.

A number of recent papers have examined the experiences of nurses working overseas, particularly those who are non-white coming to work in the UK. Their scope for career progression may be compromised: some nurses migrate in the expectation that they will work in NHS hospitals, but actually find themselves working as badly paid care assistants in nursing homes, as an overview of the experience of African nurses suggests (Likupe 2007). This has denied them the opportunity to practice the nursing (as opposed to care) skills for which they have been trained. Thus skills are under-used, expectations of the in-migrants are not met, and a potentially invaluable nurse workforce is left demoralised.

There is evidence of discrimination, racist and xenophobic attitudes (not restricted to non-white immigrants), all of which affect health and well-being. Larsen (2007) suggests a distinction between 'blatant racism', an overt hatred for, and discrimination against, minority groups, and 'aversive racism', which is more ambivalent and subtle, expressed through 'fine nuances in social interaction' (Larsen 2007: 2188). Aversive racism is a form of what Bourdieu calls symbolic violence (Crossley 2005: 319), where those who are stigmatised or devalued suffer the consequences. For Larsen, discrimination is embodied, in the sense that it impacts on the whole sense of being. One of his respondents, from Zimbabwe, considers that she is invisible in the workplace, being undermined professionally, while a male nurse from Nigeria reports that his professional skills were being constantly questioned. However, their responses (and therefore impacts on health) were quite different. While the male nurse tried to downplay the discrimination, the female nurse's personality, sense of self and plans to advance her career have been affected. Larsen regards this as a gross waste of talent, with the NHS deprived of important contributions that these nurses could be making to improve healthcare delivery in the UK.

These findings are endorsed in a similar study of overseas ethnic minority nurses employed in the NHS in southern England (Alexis et al. 2007). The theme of invisibility emerges strongly, with doctors, managers and relatives 'looking through' or disregarding these nurses. At the same time, they perceive themselves subject to surveillance. As one Indian nurse puts it: 'In this country you are followed so much you are looked at so much, you are watched so much and you are put down so much...This made me lose my confidence...it's like I had no rights' (Alexis et al. 2007: 2225). Worse, some are fearful of their jobs, in contrast to white British nurses: 'We are just careful of what we have to say, you know what I mean. They are permanent here and no matter what happens they can stay here but we are temporary nurses here and if we say something that they don't like we could be thrown out of the country' (Alexis et al. 2007: 2226).

The UK has responded to some of these concerns by establishing the Overseas Nurses Programme that provides a 20 day course taught at universities and involving placements in NHS hospitals; the mentoring provided by these organisations is aimed at enhancing the initial experiences of nurses arriving from overseas.

In some cases health professionals do not migrate but respond to emergencies or disasters across the globe. The international Red Cross was a nineteenth century response to protect and assist victims of war. More recently, Médecins Sans Frontières (MSF) was set up in 1971 by French doctors who had undertaken voluntary medical work during the Nigerian civil war (1967-70) and who rejected the neutrality shown by the Red Cross (Ticktin 2006). Rather, they saw a moral obligation to interfere and to use the mass media to lay bare the violence and suffering they witnessed first-hand. In 1980 a splinter group, Médecins du Monde (MDM), was established in response to criticism that MSF had deviated from its interventionist principles. With national sections both can be regarded as mobile transnational entities (Ticktin 2006: 123). Both have moved well beyond the provision of emergency relief to initiate long-term development projects and to campaign against injustices; thus, for example, MSF has a 'campaign for access to essential medicines' to challenge the high costs of drugs and promote research into new drug therapies to tackle neglected diseases.

Health tourism

> Bathing suit, sun block, x-rays, medical records...these may all be priorities in packing for travel to a far-flung location. (Ramirez de Arellano 2007: 193)

I want in this section to consider the international movements of individuals for the express purpose of seeking and consuming healthcare in another country.

This has become known as 'medical tourism' or 'health tourism', though despite the quotation above the motivation for seeking treatment overseas is far from recreational. Surprisingly little research has been conducted on this topic (but see Crooks et al. 2010, and Johnston et al. 2010 for useful scoping studies), though it has at times generated considerable interest in the press. One can envisage this as another aspect of globalisation (Horowitz et al. 2007). Some of what is discussed below comes from a Medical Tourism Survey undertaken in 2007 by a private company, Intuition Communication, which sponsors a web-site (www. treatmentabroad.com) offering advice to those seeking healthcare abroad.

Data from both this survey and the annual International Passenger Survey (which samples citizens leaving ports and airports) relate only to the UK. The IPS data suggest that in 2004 about 25,000 UK residents left for medical treatment abroad, but this number had grown to 77,000 in 2006. It is estimated that about 43% of these trips were for dental treatment; the paucity of provision of dental care under the NHS in the UK means that such care is increasingly expensive, especially for cosmetic treatments. Thirty per cent of trips were for cosmetic surgery, 18% for other surgery, and the remainder (less than 10%) for fertility treatment. The average spend for such treatment was about £3,700. Data suggest that savings of up to 60% on private treatment in the UK can be made when travelling to countries such as India. India is the most popular country for surgery, followed by Hungary, Poland, Turkey and Malaysia. The growing use of the internet for health-seeking information means that overseas providers can advertise readily.

There is a burgeoning demand for healthcare overseas among American citizens, with Canada and Mexico, among other countries, providing medical treatment to them. Horowitz et al. (2007) suggested that 750,000 Americans went offshore for medical treatment in 2007. The towns of Nuevo Progreso and Los Algodones in northern Mexico are described as 'dental oases attracting chartered flights full of patients from Minnesota and California in search of more affordable dental care' (Ramirez de Arellano 2007: 194).

Pressures on NHS resources, including waiting times for treatment, are likely to be a factor in seeking treatment overseas. For those with the economic means, there is an option to seek private treatment in the UK, but this will often be substantially costlier than going abroad, even allowing for the travel and subsistence costs in so doing. The same is true of the US: Horowitz and colleagues (2007) observe that the professional liability insurance premium for a surgeon in India is 1/25th that of one in New York City. In addition, overseas there is the possibility of access to treatments that are scarce, or illegal, in the domestic environment; the counter is that there may be no regulatory framework in the destination country.

Magazines, newspapers and television programmes have popularised 'body makeovers' (breast augmentation, liposuction, facelifts, and so on) and this has spawned demand for cosmetic surgery overseas, as has the ability to combine this with a vacation. Further, well-known concerns in the UK about hospital-acquired infection (such as MRSA and *Clostridium difficile*) have encouraged some to bypass domestic providers in favour of those perceived to have higher standards of hospital cleanliness. Consequently, laser eye surgery, cataract removal, knee and hip replacement, are all sought overseas. The marketing of such treatment, emphasising both quality of affordability of care, as well as the 'exoticism' of medical tourism (as Crooks et al. 2010 put it) succeeds in drawing in patients.

In reporting the results of the Medical Tourism Survey, a national newspaper recorded the views of two individuals who lauded the benefits of having done so (*Sunday Telegraph*, 28 October 2007). One man was quoted up to £24,000 to have a heart bypass operation performed privately in the UK but received this for £7,800 in the Wockhardt hospital in Delhi, India, a price that included return flights for him and his wife, 14 nights' hospital accommodation and 13 nights' recuperation at a country club. The hospital performed 500 such operations a year, more than in many UK hospitals, and had never reported a case of MRSA or *C. difficile*. The interviewee reported that 'the wards were spotless...nothing was too much trouble for the staff...there was no comparison to my treatment in Britain, where I felt like a lump of meat on the production line'. In another case a woman had travelled to Madras, India for hip 'resurfacing' (less invasive than hip replacement) and received this at a cost of £4,000, about a third of the cost in a private hospital in the UK. Crooks et al. (2010) quote a Canadian who claimed 'it's the best money I've ever spent' after returning from surgery in India. Others, such as this American patient, have to persuade their friends and families that the care is truly high quality: 'When I told people I was having surgery in Southeast Asia, some looked at me like I was crazy. They were clearly imagining me in a straw hut with someone holding fishing line and tweezers' (quoted in Crooks et al. 2010).

Of course, anecdotes such as these do not constitute detailed research evidence, as Crooks and her team (2010) have pointed out. Moreover, contrary to the above anecdotes there is evidence of possible hospital-acquired infections from, and botched operations in, overseas hospitals. The British Association of Aesthetic Plastic Surgeons have warned of the dangers of travelling overseas for cosmetic surgery, with a quarter of its members reporting increasing numbers of patients complaining of complications following surgery abroad (*The Guardian*, 18 September 2009). Others (York 2008) point to the risks of deep-vein thrombosis from long-haul flights associated with medical tourism, as discussed in Chapter 4. More recently, there is evidence of highly resistant genes (known as NDM-1) in common bacteria (such as *E. coli*), detected both in Indian patients and those who have recently returned from India after undergoing cosmetic surgery. Kumarasamy et al. (2010: 602) consider this to be an extremely serious public health problem and have advised against travel to the Indian sub-continent for corrective surgery. The authors do not mince their words: 'The potential for wider international spread...to become endemic and worldwide...is clear and frightening'.

Travelling overseas for fertility treatment ('fertility tourism', sometimes referred to as 'reproductive outsourcing': Jones and Keith 2006) has attracted some interest. In part, this is less because of the cost savings to be made and more because the law in the home country may force couples to travel overseas in order to procure fertility procedures that are restricted domestically. The Treatment Abroad website (www.treatmentabroad.net/infertility-treatment-abroad/) – 'Helping you Make the Right Choice' – lists several clinics, in Italy, Turkey, Malaya, Spain, Latvia, Hungary and Norway. The European Society for Human Reproduction and Embryology indicates that between 20-25,000 cross-border fertility treatments are carried out each year. Of British women seeking treatment abroad, over half go to the Czech Republic, where it is easier to obtain donated eggs – the reason being that in Britain donors can be paid a maximum of £250, compared with almost £500 in the Czech Republic. In addition, in Britain a child is now entitled to discover the donor's name when reaching 18 years of age, which also discourages donation. Many Italians escape legal restrictions at home by travelling to Spain for egg donation, and to Switzerland for sperm donation. French women go to Belgium for the latter. Legal restrictions are also the cause of the flow of Germans to the Czech Republic.

Recent research has questioned the lack of regulation of fertility treatment overseas. Specifically, McKelvey et al. (2009) suggest that in many countries there is no control on the number of embryos that may be transferred and that this may cause health complications, as well as additional costs to the NHS from potential multiple births. Women travelling overseas to receive fertility treatment were less likely to opt for a reduction in the number of embryos, whereas those in the UK were more likely to be counseled about the risks associated with a multiple pregnancy.

Some authors are critical of the growth of medical tourism, because of the consequences for healthcare in developing countries. Ramirez de Arellano (2007: 105) points to the example of Bumrungrad Hospital in Bangkok, Thailand, a 554-bed facility with 2600 staff (and an American management team), which treated 55,000 American patients in 2003. She suggests that this kind of infrastructure leads such countries to place a greater emphasis on technology-intensive tertiary care, at the expense of basic primary care that would benefit their own populations. 'The fact that the private health sector in Bangkok has more gamma knife, computed tomography (CT) scan, and mammography capacity than England is evidence of the distortions that occur' (Ramirez de Arellano 2007: 196). 'Islands of medical excellence' have, she argues, been created 'in a sea of medical neglect'. There are few trickle-down effects, to local populations, of having established these large private hospitals, which are invariably located in urban centres, potentially denuding rural areas of expertise. Further, she argues that it diverts medical staff otherwise employed in the public sector to work in a more lucrative private-sector setting. In contrast, others suggest that medical tourism to Asia will generate $4.4 billion in 2012, with half that amount accruing to India (Horowitz et al. 2007), and that benefits will be reaped by host countries. Also, new jobs are created within the hospitals that help boost the local economy, while incentives for medical staff employed to treat overseas visitors may slow or reverse the migration abroad of locally trained staff (as discussed in the previous section).

While there are significant international movements of people seeking health or medical care overseas, a small number seek an assisted death overseas; this is because in most countries it is illegal to assist someone to die. The legal prohibition of assisted suicide induces some to travel abroad, with the assistance of a friend or family member(s), in order to secure an end to life at the time and manner of their choosing. The Dignitas clinic in Switzerland is perhaps the most well-known venue, having assisted the deaths of almost 1000 people (the majority from Germany). Over 100 of these deaths have been of British people, some of which have become well-publicised cases because of concerns over the legal position regarding the possible prosecution of family or friends accompanying (hence assisting) them to die. The relative lack of involvement of doctors in this process (other than in prescribing the lethal drug) leads Ost (2010) to refer to this as the 'de-medicalisation' of dying.

I want to conclude this section with a brief discussion of the international organ trade, a trade sometimes referred to, not necessarily appropriately, as 'transplant tourism'. The transplantation of organs (such as kidneys) is effective in prolonging the life of those whose organs have failed. Some 66,000 kidney transplants are performed each year, in almost 100 countries. However, supply does not match demand. Thus, in Germany, for example, in 2002 there were 2325 organs donated, but 9623 patients awaiting a transplant (Hoyer 2006). Mismatch such as this, as well as the possibilities of conducting transplants between unrelated patients and donors, has led to the development of an international trade in organs. The mobilities can be of different forms, with those in need of a transplant traveling abroad, both recipients and donors travelling to a third country, or the donor being brought into a country for the operation.

Companies advertise such services on web-sites; Shimazono (2007: 956) lists several in China ($ 65-70,000 was the cost of a kidney transplant in 2007) and Pakistan, where the cost is considerably less. India has a resurgent underground market, with about 2000 Indians selling a kidney each year. The motivation of the donor is to secure resources to support families, though the additional income secured is countered by subsequent stigma and lack of employment opportunities. For the recipient, those in receipt of commercial transplants may be at risk of infections (HIV, hepatitis B: see Hoyer, 2006). Debate about the ethics of this 'trade' continues, with some (see Bakdash and Scheper-Hughes 2006) suggesting that it is hypocritical of those in the global north to reject the right of those in the global south to sell their organs. However, and quite properly, Shimazono portrays this trade as a global public health issue and suggests that the trade itself is based on structural inequality. The 'choice' to trade a kidney for cash is hardly an autonomous one, exploiting as it does the desperate circumstances of an individual.

Remote sensing: care 'at-a-distance'

Geographers and environmental scientists understand 'remote sensing' to be the use of satellites to monitor the earth's surface. Here, I appropriate the term to signify the use of modern information and communication technologies to monitor patients, but also to monitor potential disease outbreaks and to deliver healthcare in novel ways.

There is a good deal of contemporary interest among health professionals in exploring the benefits of delivering healthcare using the internet and mobile phones. Indeed, specialist journals are emerging (such as the *Journal of Medical Internet Research*) that are devoted to just these topics. So while, as we saw in the previous chapter, researchers such as Parr (2008) look at the ways in which potentially vulnerable people use the internet for social and emotional support, others are interested in more 'medicalised' encounters.

The use of information and communication technologies (ICTs) has been a feature of health and healthcare for many years, particularly in resource-rich countries. In the past 15 years the term 'telehealthcare' has emerged to encompass a set of ICTs that provide forms of health care. ('Telemedicine' is the term reserved for those applications that are distinctly medical). By *m-health* is meant the use of mobile devices (mobile phones, personal digital assistants: PDAs) to monitor, assess, and potentially improve public health.

May and his colleagues (2005) make a useful distinction between those technologies that are synchronous (thereby permitting real-time monitoring and communication) and those that are asynchronous (where exchanges of data and images are made but do not require immediate response). But my focus here is not so much on the technical apparatus involved; rather, on the ways in which the technologies are used to deliver care. May and his colleagues (2005) are interested in how the technologies form a network with other actors (health professionals, patients, and various material objects such as images). They draw on Actor Network Theory and, more generally, science and technology studies (STS) to show how people and material things combine to form networks of relations. In telemedicine, the 'actors' are not only patients and physicians, but a range of other healthcare professionals and technicians, and the material objects (recording and imaging devices) and data combine to form a broader network.

I want to describe some of the applications of these mobile technologies, at the same time reflecting critically on them. While they have undoubted benefits, they may not be the panacea for healthcare delivery that some proponents might have us believe.

One generic area of interest is in programmes that seek to provide interventions to improve health behaviours, such as smoking, alcohol consumption, and exercise. Research has looked at the effectiveness of internet assistance for helping smokers quit. Rabius et al. (2008) compared interactive internet-based cessation programmes with more static programmes that simply provided text and graphics. Participants (almost 6500 in total) were randomly assigned to different intervention and control groups. Leaving aside those who reported symptoms of depression, the results suggested that those exposed to the more interactive sites were much more likely to quit smoking than those using the static site. Other web-sites offer self-guided therapeutic interventions, for example in mental health where Cognitive Behaviour Therapy (CBT) programmes seem to be quite effective (Parr 2008: 138).

In another study Hurling and his colleagues (2007) took a group of overweight adults in the UK and assigned one to a test group with internet (and mobile phone) access and a second set had no such access. The test group received information via the internet that allowed them to consider what the barriers were to undertaking physical activity, and were given suggested solutions. Both groups were provided with wrist-worn devices to measure their activity levels but only the test group could receive emails (or phone reminders) to help plan and report levels of activity. The test group reported significantly higher levels of activity than the controls, and lost a significantly higher percentage of body fat, over the nine week period. Elkjaer and her colleagues (2010) undertook a similar study, but of people living with ulcerative colitis in Copenhagen and Dublin. Over three hundred patients were randomly assigned to either a web-group that received disease-specific information and the practical means for self-treatment, or a control group that could access routine clinic appointments. Almost 90% of patients receiving web-based care found it of value, while knowledge of the disease (hence the capacity for self-management) and quality of life improved significantly compared with controls. Patients saved time and minimised the inconvenience of travelling (often considerable) distances to clinics. From the service provider perspective, numbers of clinic visits were lower in the web group, generating modest cost savings. Studies such as these (and similar ones relating to asthma, diabetes and heart disease) suggest that web-based therapy improves the outlook for patients and may reduce healthcare costs. Further, use of the internet can help to empower patients and consumers, 'democratising' the availability of medical information and assisting people and patients 'to understand more about particular health conditions in ways potentially disruptive of traditional hierarchies in medical relationships' (Parr 2008: 137).

The key idea in applications such as these, and in telemedicine in general, is that doctors (or other health professionals) may be 'remote' and patients may be 'absent' (Mort et al. 2003). Thus a dermatologist who works in a specialist centre may be sent, over email, images of unusual skin lesions that require an expert diagnosis; the patient is not required to be co-present. The patient does not physically move, but images and emails do. This would seem to confer some benefits, not least to patients who are spared the time and cost of a potential referral to a centre many miles away. However, while distance is eroded telemedicine of this sort 'paradoxically establishes distance as a factor in a relationship previously involving direct physical touch and temporal immediacy' (Cartwright 2000: 351). Any interpersonal connections between doctor and patient that might previously have been the norm give way to relationships in which other health professionals (often nurses) act as intermediaries, thus adding a cost that cancels out others. Mort and her colleagues (2003) have examined the social dimension of telemedicine, looking in particular at the speciality of dermatology. This ought, in principle, to provide fertile ground for telemedicine, given the importance of visual inspection of skin conditions. Yet Mort and her team argue that the technology sets up new distances between doctor and patient, reducing the latter to a mere image. The patient cannot easily be herself consulted (perhaps about other symptoms and history), while the important dimension of touch is impossible. Mort suggests services and care become fragmented and are unlikely to lead to positive patient outcomes. The important human dimension to the consultation is lost. 'Both consultants operating this [dermatology] service admitted to being extremely sceptical about using it; they preferred to "see" their patients, to touch them, to talk to them, and to discuss problems with them. Dermatology, they pointed out, consists of far more than just diagnosis' (Mort et al. 2003: 287). Indeed, the service Mort describes was abandoned on the grounds it was time-consuming and not cost-effective; too many patients had to be called into the clinic for more detailed assessment.

Set against these observations, one could argue that telemedicine is 'culturally non-invasive' (Cartwright 2000: 360). For population groups such as the Canadian Inuit, those requiring care or monitoring do not have to make long journeys to be seen by non-native white Canadians; the latter may make a diagnosis but local health workers can perhaps provide any required care. Consequently, for under-served remote communities that lack health care provision telemedicine may deliver high quality care to groups previously having poor access to care.

There is, of course, no reason why these technologies are restricted to within-country care. Indeed, organisations such as the New England Medical Center, based in Boston, provide services in Latin and South America, including second opinion consultations to almost half a million paying patients in Argentina (Cartwright 2000: 365). Clearly, it is not the disadvantaged poor benefiting from this particular service. Elsewhere, profitable relationships have been established between US providers and the Middle East. For example, the Mayo Clinic, based in Minnesota, provides a telemedicine service to the United Arab Emirates, enabling the transmission of high-resolution images such as angiograms for cardiac monitoring.

Early descriptions of telehealthcare were optimistic – even exaggerated – about their transformative or utopian possibilities (the 'global clinic'). Indeed, this remains the case, with claims that new technologies will rescue stretched health service budgets, reach under-served populations, save patients time and money, help in the training of health professionals, democratise access to knowledge and thereby produce patients who are better informed about their conditions (and consequently, place fewer demands on health services). One imperative was to move towards more self-care, removing the burden (and cost) from formal health services and returning some control to people in order for them to manage their own chronic illnesses. May and his colleagues (2005: 1488) put this 'e-topian' vision very neatly as 'subtracting problems of time and space from the organization and delivery of health care'.

While Mort and her colleagues (2003) have described the transfer of work from doctors to nurses, Oudshoorn (2008) stresses a different set of concerns, relating to the redistribution of work away from the health professional and to the patient. This means that, in a telemedicine context, patients no longer enjoy productive personal relationships with their doctors. 'They have to inspect their own bodies and transmit the gathered data to healthcare professionals at telemedical centres or clinics with whom they do not have any established form of social relationship' (Oudshoorn, 2008: 273). In cardiac monitoring, the domain Oudshoorn studies, there is significant work to be done by patients in order to become competent users of these technologies. Those who trumpet telemedicine as the future of healthcare must acknowledge the work – visible and invisible – undertaken by patients and a variety of healthcare professionals, not only doctors (Oudshoorn 2009). The contrasts between face-to-face care and tele-care are summarised in Table 11.1.

Table 11.1   Contrasting co-present and telehealthcare

Face-to-face health care	Tele-healthcare
Physical proximity (co-presence)	Digital proximity
Open communication	'Protocol-driven' communication
Nurse counselling	Nurse surveillance
Care through dialogue	Care through video
Self-care as an option	Self-care as an obligation
Contextualised care	Individualised care

Source: Based on Oudshoorn (2009): 402.

Having considered the social dimensions of telemedicine and telehealthcare, what of their effectiveness? Deshpande et al. (2009) reviewed over 50 studies of asynchronous telehealth; that is, those that have captured data (video, images and so on) and transmitted these for subsequent interpretation at a remote site. The majority of studies the authors reviewed were in dermatology. Overall, these studies showed evidence of high levels of diagnostic accuracy, reduced waiting times, fewer unnecessary referrals, and reduced in-person visits. Many of the studies noted high levels of satisfaction among patients and health professionals, suggesting that the critiques by Mort, May and their colleagues, outlined above, are possibly unfounded.

I want to turn now to consider applications of m-health; the applications of technologies such as mobile phones and personal digital assistants (PDAs) in capturing and transmitting health data.

Using such new technologies data can be obtained quickly and efficiently in the field and in real-time. This has clear advantages over paper-based surveys that subsequently require manual data entry. There are many examples, including the tracking of mosquito-borne dengue fever in Brazil, where time spent gathering GPS data on the locations of water sources and disease cases is substantially reduced. An advanced economy example is given by Cooper and colleagues (2008), seeking to track the spatial diffusion of influenza (and norovirus) across the UK. Their study uses data obtained from NHS Direct, a national database generated by calls to an advice line. Those calls, over a 12 month period, relating to high fever and vomiting were extracted and referenced geographically, permitting the authors to map and analyse the data for significant space-time clusters of cases. This form of synchronous telehealth provides the potential for an early warning system to monitor disease outbreaks and spread. Cartwright (2000: 352-4) gives the example of the Ebola outbreak in the former Zaire in 1995. Here, a physician suspected a patient of carrying the virus and immediately called the Centers for Disease Control (CDC) in Atlanta with a description of symptoms and later sending samples. The disease was confirmed in Atlanta, not locally. 'Together the various technologies of imaging and telecommunications are employed to collapse distances with the reciprocal aims of containing crises in "remote" regions and protecting health at home' (Cartwright, 2000: 353).

At a much broader, international scale there are a number of projects and sites devoted to real-time (or near real-time) surveillance of disease outbreaks, culling data from different sources to generate public health intelligence. A good example is 'HealthMap' (www.healthmap.org), an interactive system that highlights disease outbreaks in different parts of the world. Other researchers suggest that search engines such as Google can be exploited; thus, logs of keywords can potentially be used to highlight disease outbreaks. For example, mining the web for searches of 'swine flu' might help detect local outbreaks (Ginsberg et al. 2009).

The Vodafone Foundation has produced a comprehensive report on uses of mobile technology for healthcare in the developing world (Vital Wave Consulting 2009). The report suggests that 64% of all mobile phone users are found in the global south, and that the growing ubiquity of mobile phones is a key platform for expanding mobile technologies for health. Such access to mobile phones contrasts with other technologies and with health infrastructure.

Short message service (SMS) offers a cost-effective and extremely efficient vehicle for transmitting messages designed to influence behaviour. SMS is popular, unobtrusive and offers confidentiality, and it can be used for either one-way alerts or for interactivity. PDAs and other devices can be used for the remote monitoring of patients rather than requiring their attendance at a fixed facility such as a health centre or hospital. Evidence from South Africa (the SIMpill project) suggests that TB patients with mobile phones, when reminded by healthcare workers (themselves former TB patients) to take medication, generated 90% compliance after this initiative was introduced, compared with less than 60% before the intervention (Vital Wave Consulting (2009: 16). Project Masiluleke in South Africa sends over 1 million SMS messages a day encouraging mobile phone users to contact HIV and TB call centres. Trained operators then provide accurate healthcare information, counselling, and referrals to local testing clinics. It is envisaged that the programme will eventually include anti-retroviral therapy support and at-home HIV testing. In Uganda an SMS-based, interactive, multiple choice quiz (the Text to Change programme) was administered to over 15,000 mobile phone users in rural areas as a vehicle for promoting HIV awareness and encouraging testing. It led to a 40% increase in people seeking an HIV test. Lester and his colleagues (2010) demonstrated significant improvements in adherence to therapy for HIV patients in Kenya, among those who had access to SMS. Equally convincingly, those patients who were given access to SMS also subsequently demonstrated significantly greater suppression of viral load compared with a control group. SMS was used here to encourage patients to take antiretroviral therapy (ART) and to provide additional support. Patients were invited to respond to the SMS as to whether they were feeling well or had a problem (in which case they were called by a clinician). As the authors note, SMS is inexpensive and effective given the near-ubiquitous use of mobile phones. Travel costs for patients are saved, and in areas where travel is not always straightforward, any intervention at-a-distance that proves to be clinically effective is to be welcomed. Of course, an issue is whether the programmes of activity are maintained over a longer period. Nonetheless, the results are suggestive of the value of mobile phone-based interventions, coupled perhaps with internet support.

More directly, the phones themselves can have chips inserted that can take and transmit a saliva or urine sample that is analysed remotely for sexual infections (STIs) and a result returned to the sender, along with advice as to where to go for treatment if the result is positive (*Guardian* newspaper, 6 November 2010). The public health aspiration is to reduce the STIs (currently almost half a million diagnosed each year), and this may provide more rapid diagnosis, obviating the need for a potentially embarrassing direct clinical consultation.

The Vodafone report referred to above calls for 'large-scale evidence of mHealth effectiveness, as measure by long-term, repeatable improved outcomes in either health or economic terms' (Vital Wave Consulting (2009: 17). Indeed, this imperative would seem essential as a means of assessing telehealthcare in general. But, as noted above, the technologies themselves cannot be divorced from the communities of human actors, whether patients, carers or health professionals. May and colleagues (2005) paint a sober picture of telemedicine, suggesting that its hopes remain unfulfilled. They contrast this with quite conventional technologies, such as the provision of advice (as opposed to *care*) over the telephone. Those systems that deliver information may work, but those providing diagnosis and disease management have yet to prove their worth.

One vision for the near future is for people to have access to their personal health record through their mobile phone (Lefebvre 2009). Lefebvre argues that mobile technologies serve to develop and expand relationships between producers and consumers of healthcare, and they become marketing tools as much as communications devices. 'In this world, the language of search, proximity, recommendation, links, discovery, and the currency of information become the essence of new approaches to addressing issues of equity, civic engagement, poverty, health, and harnessing our collective intelligence to improve the public's health and well-being' (Lefebvre 2009: 494).

Concluding remarks

Some of the mobilities which I have discussed here are an embodiment of globalisation. Health professionals are competing in a global labour market, while the relative ease of international travel and the creation of niche providers (in the global south) to address health care demands in the global north is another marker of globalisation. But these mobilities bring with them potential or real inequalities. Medical tourism risks denuding some regions of valuable expertise if trained staff leave those areas to cater for a different clientele in hospitals providing care for those from abroad. It may also serve to perpetuate health inequalities in the 'sender' countries, since the costs of overseas care may be considerable, and affordable only by those with the material resources to seek it out. While it would be an exaggeration to say that such care is accessible only to a kinetic elite, it is true that this particular form of mobility excludes many. Those that do avail themselves of such care may lay themselves open to risks of infection that have to be dealt with upon return.

From a Foucauldian perspective one could take telemedicine as a form of surveillance at a distance, where either individual bodies or groups of people are monitored, scrutinised, recorded, and results stored for immediate or subsequent analysis. An alternative view would be to regard it as a panacea, a means of delivering healthcare effectively and efficiently, benefiting both the patient and over-stretched healthcare systems and budgets. Almost inevitably, the truth lies somewhere in-between. What can be said with confidence is that the applications of 'virtual mobilities of care' will explode in the near future and that much of what has been presented in this chapter will date rapidly. New technologies will emerge to supersede those presently on the market and – one imagines – these will become more ubiquitous, reaching many more as mobile communications networks expand further. But the technologies are merely one component; human actors, whether health professionals or lay people, need to be convinced that they have enduring value.

Chapter 12

Conclusions: Emerging Themes for Mobilities and Health

The focus in this book has been on the relationships between mobilities and health, relationships that can be health-promoting but also not conducive to good health and well-being. As I have suggested, at times some of these mobilities have negative consequences for those *who do not move*; for example, those living near busy major airports, or along heavily trafficked streets, or those exploited by tourists. The immobile live in places that are impacted by the activities of the mobile. But the mobile too inhabit places that may affect their health and well-being, either positively or negatively. Places will always be settings that have significant contextual effects on health, well-being, and disease, and geographers, epidemiologists and other (social) scientists will continue to describe, and explain, these relationships. Mobilities and networks matter, but so too do places.

In this final chapter I consider, first, some mobilities trends and the extent to which we might 'rein in' mobility, whether for the good of the planet or the good of our health (hardly independent imperatives, of course). Links to the sustainability agenda are considered briefly, in an examination of the inter-relationships between mobilities and climate change. These relationships demand further theoretical and empirical excavation that is beyond the scope of the present book.

Mobilities trends and implications for human health

The increasing widespread availability of new mobile technologies – mobile phones, the internet, and now social networking – suggests that the connectivity these resources offer might obviate the need for frequent travel. It certainly seems to obviate the need for letter-writing; only 25 years ago one kept in touch with friends overseas with a letter that might have taken several days to arrive. Now the contact can be a constant one via Facebook or Twitter, and a whole network of friends is instantly up to date. Whether these ephemera are better vehicles for maintaining the health and well-being (of the recipients) than direct meetings and material correspondence is an issue for further research. For the sender, there may be value in their being able to assert their identity and presence in cyber-space.

To what extent does this kind of virtual travel substitute for trip-making, offering savings in time, money and (an increasing concern) environmental damage? Virtual mobility may turn out to be a very compelling response to the need to reduce carbon footprints. Kaufmann and Montulet (2008: 48) suggest that 'people try to reduce the impact of their moves on their lives, their social networks, their anchoring, while at the same time attempting to achieve maximum moving potential – motility – in order to respond to the mobility injunction that characterises contemporary Western societies'.

If we are serious about addressing the perceived negative consequences of mobility for human health then new environmental policies need better promotion, funding, and adoption. These include: further measures to control vehicle exhaust emissions; improved public transport; speed restrictions on roads; increasing taxes on car use and fuel consumption; and improved facilities for bicycle users. Measures such as these will improve population health, as well as the health of individuals. These mean reducing our dependence on oil that has fuelled growth over many decades.

Such issues have been addressed by several authors. In an explicitly African context, Gordon Pirie has asked whether, in the development of the continent, it has to be the case that transport investment and subsequent mobility are pre-requisites for growth. This is a question of moral economy; why should we deprive one major global region the opportunities for growth and development that the global north has enjoyed for 150 years? Pirie's answer is quite clear: 'Even in the African situation of a pent up desire for increased mobility, there may be considerable dividends from *restraining* mobility, if not through public policy, then through social and personal lifestyle choice' (Pirie 2009: 28, my italics). We should, he argues, curb expectations and avoid merely duplicating Western mobility histories by default. Indeed, he coins the term 'slowbility' to highlight the plea for us to forego the quest for ever-increasing accessibility and increased levels of motorisation and its associated infrastructure. He would prefer to see this replaced with 'virtual e-mobility' and 'virtuous physical mobility' (by which he means sustainable transport: Pirie 2009: 32). This has echoes of Bergmann's (2008a) plea to rediscover slowness. Such a rediscovery, and a reduction in travel that continues to add to carbon footprints, could help reduce the impact of mobility on climate change, with potential health benefits. It is to climate change that I now turn briefly.

Impacts of mobilities on climate change, and of climate change on mobilities

Surely one of the most pressing issues for those interested in the intersection of mobilities and health is to outline the likely consequences of climate change for human movement. As mean temperatures continue to rise in particular parts of the world, can we trace the effects this will have? What do we know about human movement as a result of sea-level rises or crop failures due to climate change?

Let us be clear about the contributions made by transport to climate change. Data from the UK suggest that transport contributes about 44 million tonnes of carbon emissions each year, three-quarters of these emissions coming from road transport (Table 13.1); this is broadly in line with data for Europe as a whole

Table 12.1   Transport-related emissions of CO$_2$ in the UK (millions of tonnes)

Source	2003	Per cent
Passenger cars	19.8	45.2
Light-duty (vans etc)	4.4	10.0
Buses	1.0	2.3
Heavy goods (trucks etc)	7.2	16.4
Motorcycles	0.1	0.2
Railways	0.3	0.7
Domestic air transport	0.6	1.4
International air transport	8.1	18.5
Domestic shipping	0.9	2.1
International shipping	1.4	3.2
Total	43.8	100.0

Source: Potter and Bailey (2008: 34)

(Potter and Bailey 2008). The contribution from public transport on the road is minor in relation to that from cars and trucks. Note that rail travel generates under 1% of transport-related emissions. Air travel accounts for 20% of emissions. Potter and Bailey (2008: 35) note that international air travel is excluded from the Kyoto Protocol on global climate change (1997) because of the problems involved in determining which country should be assigned the emissions.

In an attempt to limit this burden of pollution there are several initiatives that can be taken. One, adopted by some towns and cities, is to recognise 'car-free days', where motorists are invited to relinquish their cars for a day in order to encourage walking, cycling and the use of buses. September 22nd is now recognised as 'World Car Free Day', and while this has yet to be adopted other than by a few enthusiasts local events have been held in recent years in Washington DC, Jakarta (Indonesia), Toronto and several Dutch cities.

There is a strong, emerging literature on the potential impacts of global climate change on human health (see, for example, the overview in Gatrell and Elliott 2009, Chapter 9). Mobility contributes to global climate change, which itself has health consequences, but there are feedback loops, inasmuch as climate change will affect mobility, in part as potentially large population groups seek to relocate to cooler climates. Yet this literature is relatively silent on the consequences for population movement and little has been achieved beyond developing rather simple conceptual models. For example, McLeman and Smit (2006) suggest that the potential for migration depends both upon degree of exposure to climate change and on the capacity of individuals or communities to adapt to this. They acknowledge that it also depends upon economic and political constraints and on the availability of capital to enable a move or to adapt locally. Perch-Nielsen et al. (2008) develop this further. Flooding can be caused by tropical cyclones and by increased precipitation, as well as by sea level rise. Consequences of flooding will include direct effects, such as drowning of people and animals, and loss of homes. More indirect effects will include loss of land for cultivation, damage to crops and livestock, as well as contamination of food and water supplies. Employment will suffer and the incidence of disease will increase. People will be forced from their homes, as unwilling migrants. We witnessed all these effects in the devastating floods in Pakistan in summer 2010.

These conceptual sketches are starting points, but we need to move beyond these and develop case studies. Such case studies as there are focus on migration following hurricanes and other natural disasters (as we saw in Chapter 6) and suggest there is considerable return migration after the event. But in the case of long-term climate change the likelihood of return migration seems questionable. What we need are some simulations of possible outcomes. As a geographer, I would want to know the probable sources of migrants and their possible destinations, so that contingency plans can be explored to deal with possible large influxes. How far will people move, how will moves be socially patterned, and what resources will be in place to help? As we saw in Chapter 6 refugees go to great lengths to seek a better life in (for example) Europe and we can only speculate that 'environmental' refugees will be at least as desperate.

Journey's end

Plenty of evidence has been presented in this book to support claims that mobility is of benefit for human health. Travel itself, as well as what awaits the trip, can be liberating and pleasurable, particularly when it is sufficiently slow to permit enjoyment of the journey without undue delay. If trips involve physical exercise, they can help maintain or improve physical health. But, as also evidenced in earlier chapters, mobilities can be damaging of one's own health and of others'. It can be a risky business. Such risks include exposure to environmental pollution and accidents during the trip, with further risks awaiting the traveller at the destination if sufficient care is not taken. However, while the risk society involves risks for the mobile, the risks are socially patterned and unequally distributed. For example, road traffic 'accidents' (crashes) appear to impact more on the relatively disadvantaged, while, at the extreme, those who are fleeing persecution, disaster, or 'development' imposed by remote governments or organisations encounter risks that are of a very different order of magnitude. Some people are forced to move, and others may be impacted adversely by the movements of others.

Both benefits and risks are affected by the volume and velocity of transport and communications. Places continue to converge in time-space, and this convergence opens up new possibilities for the mobilities of both people and (potentially) infections. Growing volumes of air traffic, and better connections between cities, all serve to create new globalising networks that structure flow and disease spread and contribute to the world risk society identified by Ulrich Beck. Again, however, it would be foolish to ignore the positives in these network structures. Movement brings new interactions that can build network capital to enrich human life. We do indeed live in a networked society, connected by transport and communication networks that bring people together, whether in real space or cyber-space. We can be quite certain that social relations and structures in cyber-space will continue to develop in ways that may yet be themselves uncertain or unknown. Many of these will perhaps help deliver health and social care in new and important contexts. What we can be certain of is that commentators will continue to debate the merits of such technological engagements, with some (notably, Sherry Turkle 2011) worrying that we may be 'alone together' in our movements around cyber-space.

I end this book where I started, namely with an exhortation for geographers interested in health to engage more than they have done in studying health and well-being on the move; and for those interested in mobilities to address their neglect of the relations between mobilities and health. Scientists and social scientists interested in a genuinely inter-disciplinary perspective on public health ought to find much to provoke and intrigue them if they pursue this agenda.

Bibliography

Aagaard-Hansen, J., Nombela, N. and Alvar, J. 2010. Population movement: a key factor in the epidemiology of neglected tropical diseases. *Tropical Medicine and International Health*, 1, 1281-8.

Abramson, D., Stehling-Ariza, T., Garfield, R. and Redlener, I. 2008. Prevalence and predictors of mental health distress post-Katrina: findings from the Gulf Coast Child and Family Health Study. *Disaster Medicine and Public Health Preparedness*, 2, 77-86.

Abu-habib, L. 1998. The use and abuse of female domestic workers from Sri Lanka in Lebanon. *Gender & Development*, 6, 52-6.

Adams, J. 2005. *Risk*. London: Routledge.

Adams, V., van Hattum, T. and English, D. 2009. Chronic disaster syndrome: displacement, disaster capitalism, and the eviction of the poor from New Orleans. *American Ethnologist*, 36, 615-36.

Adey, P. 2010. *Mobility*. London: Routledge.

Adey, P., Budd, L. and Hubbard, P. 2007. Flying lessons: exploring the social and cultural geographies of global air travel. *Progress in Human Geography*, 31, 773-91.

Agredano, Y.Z., Chan, J.L., Kimball, R.C. and Kimball, A.B. 2006. Accessibility to air travel correlates strongly with increasing melanoma incidence. *Melanoma Research*, 16, 77-81.

Agudelo-Suárez, A., Gil-González, D., Ronda-Pérez, E., Porthé, V. and others. 2009. Discrimination, work and health in immigrant populations in Spain, *Social Science & Medicine*, 68, 1866-74.

Ahmed, Q.A., Arabi, Y.M. and Memish, Z.A. 2006. Health risks at the Hajj. *Lancet*, 367, 1008-15.

Aitchison, C., MacLeod, N.E. and Shaw, S.J. 2000. *Leisure and Tourism Landscapes: Social and Cultural Geographies*. London: Routledge.

Alden, D. and Miller, J.C. 1987. Out of Africa: the slave trade and the transmission of smallpox to Brazil, 1560-1831. *Journal of Interdisciplinary History*, 18, 195-224.

Aldrich, T.K., Gustave, J., Hall, G.B., Cohen, H.W. and others. 2010. Lung function in rescue workers at the World Trade Center after 7 years. *New England Journal of Medicine*, 362, 1263-72.

Alexis, O., Vydelingum, V. and Robbins, I. 2007. Engaging with a new reality: experiences of overseas minority ethnic nurses in the NHS. *Journal of Clinical Nursing*, 16, 2221-8.

Ali, S.H. 2008. SARS as an emergent complex: toward a networked approach to urban infectious disease, in *Networked Disease: Emerging Infections in the Global City*, edited by S.H. Ali and R. Keil. Chichester: Wiley-Blackwell.

Ali, S.H. and Keil, R. 2008. *Networked Disease: Emerging Infections in the Global City*. Chichester: Wiley-Blackwell.

Anbesse, B., Hanlon, C., Alem, A., Packer, S. and Whitley, R. 2009. Migration and mental health: a study of low-income Ethiopian women working in Middle Eastern countries. *International Journal of Social Psychiatry*, 55, 557-68.

Anderson, J. 2010. Treat with care: Africans and HIV in the UK, in *Mobility, Sexuality and AIDS*, edited by F. Thomas, M. Haour-Knipe and P. Aggleton. London: Routledge.

Anderson, N. 1961. *The Hobo: The Sociology of the Homeless Man*. Chicago: University of Chicago Press (reprint of 1923 monograph).

Arnold, D. 1993. Social crisis and epidemic disease in the famines of nineteenth-century India. *Social History of Medicine*, 6, 385-404.

Azara, A., Piana, A., Sotgiu, G., Dettori, M. and others. 2006. Prevalence study of Legionella spp. contamination in ferries and cruise ships. *BMC Public Health* doi: 10.1186/1471-2458-6-100.

Baehr, P. 2008. City under siege: authoritarian toleration, mask culture, and the SARS crisis in Hong Kong, in *Networked Disease: Emerging Infections in the Global City*, edited by S.H. Ali and R. Keil. Chichester: Wiley-Blackwell.

Baig, F., Hameed, M.A., Li, M., Shorthouse, G., Roalfe, A.K. and Daley, A. 2009. Association between active commuting to school, weight and physical activity status in ethnically diverse adolescents predominantly living in deprived communities. *Public Health*, 123, 39-41.

Baiju, D.S. and James, L.A. 2003. Parachuting: a sport of chance and expense. *Injury*, 34, 215-17.

Bakdash, T. and Scheper-Hughes, N. 2006. Is it ethical for patients with renal disease to purchase kidneys from the world's poor? *PLoS Medicine*, 3, doi: 10.1371/journal.pmed.0030349.

Baumert, J., Erazo, N. and Ladwig, K.H. 2005. Ten-year incidence and time trends of railway suicides in Germany from 1991 to 2000. *European Journal of Public Health*, 16, 173-8.

Beck, U. 1992. *Risk Society*. London: Sage.

Behrentz, E., Sabin, L.D., Winder, A.M., Fitz, D.R. and others. 2005. Relative importance of school bus-related microenvironments to children's pollutant exposure. *Journal of Air Waste Management Association*, 55, 1418-30.

Bennett, G.G., McNeill, L.H., Wolin, K.Y., Duncan, D.T., Puleo, E. and Emmons, KM. 2007. Safe to walk? Neighborhood safety and physical activity among public housing residents. *PLoS Medicine*, 4, 1599-606.

Bentham, G. 1988. Migration and morbidity: implications for geographical studies of disease. *Social Science & Medicine*, 26, 49-54.

Bernardo, J. 2007. Tuberculosis, in *Immigrant Medicine*, edited by P.F. Walker and E.D. Barnett. Philadelphia: Elsevier.

Bergmann, S. 2008a. The beauty of speed or the discovery of slowness – why do we need to rethink mobility? in *The Ethics of Mobilities: Rethinking Place, Exclusion, Freedom and Environment*, edited by S. Bergmann and T. Sager. Farnham: Ashgate.

Bergmann, S. 2008b. The beauty of speed or the cross of mobility? Introductory reflections on the aesth/ethics of space, justice and motion, in *Spaces of Mobility*, edited by S. Bergmann, T. Hoff and T. Sager. London: Equinox.

Beyrer, C. 2004. Global child trafficking. *Lancet*, 364, 16-17.

Bhalla, K., Naghavi, M., Shahraz, S., Bartels, D. and Murray, C.J.L. 2009. Building national estimates of the burden of road traffic injuries in developing countries from all available data sources: Iran. *Injury Prevention*, 15, 150-6.

Bharti, N., Djibo, A., Ferrari, M.J., Grais, R.F. and others. 2010. Measles hotspots and epidemiological connectivity. *Epidemiology and Infection*, 138, 1308-16.

Biemann, U. 2002. Touring, routing and trafficking female geobodies, in *Mobilizing Place, Placing Mobility*, edited by G. Verstraete and T. Cresswell. Amsterdam: Rodopi.

Bischoff, A., Schneider, M., Denhaerynck, K. and Battegay, E. 2009. Health and ill health of asylum seekers in Switzerland: an epidemiological study. *European Journal of Public Health*, 19, 59-64.

Bissell, D. 2008. Visualising everyday geographies: practices of vision through travel-time, *Transactions, Institute of British Geographers*, 34, 42-60.

Bissell, D. 2009a. Conceptualising differently-mobile passengers: geographies of everyday encumbrance in the railway station. *Social & Cultural Geography*, 10, 173-94.

Bissell, D. 2009b. Moving with others: the sociality of the railway journey, in *The Cultures of Alternative Mobilities: Routes Less Travelled*, edited by P. Vannini. Farnham: Ashgate.

Borges, G., Breslau, J., Su, M., Miller, M., Medina-Mora, M.E. and Aguilar-Gaxiola, S. 2009. Immigration and suicidal behaviour among Mexicans and Mexican Americans. *American Journal of Public Health*, 99, 728-33.

Bossak, B.H. and Welford, M.R. 2009. Did medieval trade activity and a viral etiology control the spatial extent and seasonal distribution of Black Death mortality? *Medical Hypotheses*, 72, 749-52.

Bostock, L. 2001. Pathways of disadvantage? Walking as a mode of transport among low-income mothers. *Health and Social Care in the Community*, 9, 11-18.

Bourque, L.B., Siegel, J.M., Kano, M. and Wood, M.M. 2006. Weathering the storm: the impact of hurricanes on physical and mental health. *Annals, American Academy of Political and Social Science*, 604, 129-51.

Boyle, P. and Norman, P. 2010. Migration and health, in *A Companion to Health and Medical Geography*, edited by T. Brown, S. McLafferty and G. Moon. Oxford: Wiley-Blackwell.

Bradley, D.E. and van Willigen, M. 2010. Migration and psychological well-being among older adults: a growth curve analysis based on panel data from the

Health and Retirement Study, 1996-2006. *Journal of Aging and Health*, 20, 1-32.

Braun, B. 2008. Thinking the city through SARS: bodies, topologies, politics, in *Networked Disease: Emerging Infections in the Global City*, edited by S.H. Ali and R. Keil. Chichester: Wiley-Blackwell.

Briggs, D.J., de Hoogh, K., Morris, C. and Gulliver, J. 2008. Effects of travel mode on exposures to particulate air pollution. *Environment International*, 34, 12-22.

Brown, R.P.C. and Connell, J. 2004. The migration of doctors and nurses from South Pacific Island Nations. *Social Science & Medicine*, 58, 2193-2210.

Brown, T., McLafferty, S. and Moon, G. 2010. *A Companion to Health and Medical Geography*. Oxford: Wiley-Blackwell.

Brush, B.L. and Sochalski, J. 2007. International nurse migration: lessons from the Philippines. *Policy, Politics, and Nursing Practice*, 8, 37-46.

Budd, L. 2009. The view from the air: the cultural geographies of flight, in *The Cultures of Alternative Mobilities: Routes Less Travelled*, edited by P. Vannini. Farnham: Ashgate.

Budd, L., Bell, M. and Brown, T. 2009. Of plagues, planes and politics: controlling the global spread of infectious diseases by air. *Political Geography*, 28, 426-35.

Cairney, J. and Ostbye, T. 1999. Time since immigration and excess body weight. *Canadian Journal of Public Health*, 90, 120-4.

Cairncross, F. 1997. *The Death of Distance: How the Communications Revolution Will Change Our Lives*. Cambridge, Mass: Harvard Business School Press.

Camlin, C.S., Hosegood, V., Newell, M-L., McGrath, N. and others. 2010. Gender, migration and HIV in rural KwaZulu-Natal, South Africa. *PLoS One*, 5, doi: 10.1371/journal.pone.0011539.

Cantor-Graae, E. and Selten, J-P. 2005. Schizophrenia and migration: a meta-analysis and review. *American Journal of Psychiatry*, 162, 12-24.

Canzler, W. 2008. The paradoxical nature of automobility, in *Tracing Mobilities: Towards a Cosmopolitan Perspective*, edited by W. Canzler, V. Kaufmann and S. Kesselring. Farnham: Ashgate.

Canzler, W., Kaufmann, V. and Kesselring, S. 2008. *Tracing Mobilities: Towards a Cosmopolitan Perspective*, Farnham: Ashgate.

Cao, Y., Hwang, S-S. and Xi, J. 2008. Project-induced migration, secondary stressors, and health: a panel analysis of migrants of the Three Gorges Dam Project, China, paper delivered at Annual Meeting of the American Sociological Association, Boston, Mass. Available at: www.allacademic.com/meta/p243024_index.html.

Cartwright, L. 2000. Reach out and heal someone: telemedicine and the globalization of health care. *Health*, 4, 347-77.

Chakrabati, R. 2010. Therapeutic networks of pregnancy care: Bengali immigrant women in New York City. *Social Science & Medicine*, 71, 362-9.

Chisholm, J.F. 2006. Cyberspace violence against girls and adolescent females. *Annals, New York Academy of Sciences*, 1087, 74-89.

Christakis, N.A. and Fowler, J.H. 2009. *Connected: The Amazing Power of Social Networks and How they Shape our Lives*. London: HarperCollins.

Christakos, G., Olea, R.A. and Yu, H-L. 2007. Recent results on the spatiotemporal modelling and comparative analysis of Black Death and bubonic plague epidemics. *Public Health*, 121, 700-20.

Claassen, C.A., Carmody, T., Stewart, S.M., Bossarte, R.M. and others. 2010. Effect of 11 September 2001 terrorist attacks in the USA on suicide in areas surrounding the crash sites, *British Journal of Psychiatry*. 196, 359-64.

Clark, B.R., Ferketich, A.K., Fisher, J.L. Ruymann, F.B. and others. 2007. Evidence of population mixing based on the geographical distribution of childhood leukemia in Ohio. *Pediatric Blood & Cancer*, 49, 797-802.

Clark, C., Martin, R., van Kempen, E., Alfred, T. and others. 2006. Exposure- effect relations between aircraft and road traffic noise exposure at school and reading comprehension: the RANCH project. *American Journal of Epidemiology*, 163, 27-37.

Clark, C., Kawachi, I., Ryan, L. Ertel, K. and others. 2009. Perceived neighbourhood safety and incident mobility disability among elders: the hazards of poverty. *BMC Public Health*, 9, doi: 10.1186/1471-2458-9-162.

Clarke, M. 1994. Railway suicide in England and Wales, 1850-1949. *Social Science & Medicine,* 38, 401-7.

Clarke, R.V. and Poyner, B. 1994. Preventing suicide on the London Underground. *Social Science & Medicine*, 38, 443-6.

Clemens, M.A. and Pettersson, G. 2008. New data on African health professionals abroad. *Human Resources for Health*, 6, 1478-91.

Cliff, A.D., Haggett, P. and Ord, J.K. 1986. *Spatial Aspects of Influenza Epidemics*. London: Pion.

Cliff, A.D., Haggett, P. and Smallman-Raynor, M.R. 1998. *Deciphering Global Epidemics: Analytic Approaches to the Disease Records of World Cities*, 1888-1912. Cambridge: Cambridge University Press.

Cliff, A.D., Haggett, P. and Smallman-Raynor, M.R. 2000. *Island Epidemics*, Oxford: Oxford University Press.

Cliff, A.D., Smallman-Raynor, M.R., Haggett, P., Stroup, D.F. and Thacker, S.B. 2009. *Infectious Diseases, Emergence and Re-Emergence: a Geographical Analysis*. Oxford: Oxford University Press.

Clingingsmith, D., Khwaja, A.I. and Kremer, M. 2008. Estimating the impact of the Hajj: religion and tolerance in Islam's global gathering. *Kennedy School of Government*, Harvard University, RWP08-022.

Cohen, B.S., Bronzaft, A.L., Heikkinen, M., Goodman, J. and Nadas, A. 2008. Airport-related air pollution and noise. *Journal of Occupational and Environmental Hygiene*, 5, 119-29.

Coker, R. and Ingram, A. 2006. Passports and pestilence: migration, security and contemporary border control of infectious diseases, in *Medicine at the*

Border: Disease, Globalization and Security, 1850 to the Present, edited by A. Bashford. Basingstoke: Palgrave Macmillan.

Collins, D. and Kearns, R.A. 2010. Walking school buses in the Auckland region: a longitudinal assessment. *Transport Policy*, 17, 1-8.

Conradson, D. 2005. Freedom, space and perspective: moving encounters with other ecologies, in *Emotional Geographies*, edited by J. Davidson, L. Bondi and M. Smith. Farnham: Ashgate.

Convery, I., Welshman, J. and Bashford, A. 2006. Where is the border? Screening for tuberculosis in the United Kingdom and Australia, 1950-2000, in *Medicine at the Border: Disease, Globalization and Security, 1850 to the Present*, edited by A. Bashford. Basingstoke: Palgrave Macmillan.

Convery, I., Mort, M., Baxter, J. and Bailey, C. 2008. *Animal Disease and Human Trauma: Emotional Geographies of Disaster*. Basingstoke: Palgrave Macmillan.

Cook, N.D. 1988. *Born to Die: Disease and New World Conquest, 1492-1650*. Cambridge: Cambridge University Press.

Cooper, A.R., Page, A.S., Wheeler, B.W., Griew, P. and others. 2010. Mapping the walk to school using accelerometry combined with a Global Positioning System. *American Journal of Preventive Medicine*, 38, 178-83.

Cooper, D.L., Smith, G.E., Regan, M., Large, S. and Groenewegen, P.P. 2008. Tracking the spatial diffusion of influenza and norovirus using telehealth data: a spatiotemporal analysis of syndromic data. *BMC Medicine*, 6, doi: 10.1186/1741-7015-6-16.

Couclelis, H. 2009. Rethinking time geography in the information age. *Environment and Planning A*, 41, 1556-75.

Craddock, S. 2008. Tuberculosis and the anxieties of containment, in *Networked Disease: Emerging Infections in the Global City*, edited by S.H. Ali and R. Keil. Chichester: Wiley-Blackwell.

Craig, G.M. 2007. Nation, migration and tuberculosis. *Social Theory and Health*, 5, 267-84.

Cramer, E.H., Blanton, C.J., Blanton, L.H., Vaughan, G.H. and others. 2006. Epidemiology of gastroenteritis on cruise ships, 2001-2004. *American Journal of Preventive Medicine*, 30, 252-7.

Crang, M. 2002. Commentary: between places – producing hubs, flows, and networks. *Environment and Planning A*, 34, 569-74.

Cresswell, T. 1997. Weeds, plagues, and bodily secretions: a geographical interpretation of metaphors of displacement. *Annals, Association of American Geographers*, 87, 330-45.

Cresswell, T. 2001. *The Tramp in America*. London: Reaktion Books.

Cresswell, T. 2002. Introduction: theorizing place, in *Mobilizing Place, Placing Mobility*, edited by G. Verstraete and T. Cresswell. Amsterdam: Rodopi.

Cresswell, T. 2006. *On the Move: Mobility in the Modern Western World*. London: Routledge.

Crooks, V.A., Kingsbury, P., Snyder, J. and Johnston, R. 2010. What is known about the patient's experience of medical tourism? A scoping review. *BMC Health Services Research*, 10, doi: 10.1186/1472-6963-10-266.

Crossley, N. 2005. *Key Concepts in Critical Social Theory*. London: Sage.

Crowley, C. 2009. The mental health needs of refugee children: a review of literature and implications for nurse practitioners. *Journal of the American Academy of Nurse Practitioners*, 21, 322-31.

Cummins, S., Curtis, S., Diez-Roux, A.V. and Macintyre, S. 2007. Understanding and representing 'place' in health research: a relational approach, *Social Science & Medicine*, 65, 1825-38.

Cunningham, S.A., Ruben, J.D. and Narayan, K.M.V. 2008. Health of foreign-born people in the United States: a review. *Health & Place*, 14, 623-35.

Curson, P. and McCracken, K. 2006. An Australian perspective of the 1918-1919 influenza pandemic. *New South Wales Public Health Bulletin*, 17, 103-7.

Curtis, S. 2010. *Space, Place and Mental Health*. Farnham: Ashgate.

Cutts, B.B., Darby, K.J., Boone, C.G. and Brewis, A. 2009. City structure, obesity, and environmental justice: an integrated analysis of physical and social barriers to walkable streets and park access. *Social Science & Medicine*, 69, 1314-22.

Davidson, J., Smith, M. and Bondi, L. 2007. *Emotional Geographies*. Farnham: Ashgate.

Davies, G. and Whyatt, D. 2009. A least-cost approach to personal exposure reduction. *Transactions in GIS*, 13, 229-46.

Davies, S.E. 2008. Securitizing infectious disease. *International Affairs*, 84: 295-313.

Deane, K.D., Parkhurst, J., and Johnston, D. 2010. Linking migration, mobility and HIV. *Tropical Medicine and International Health*, 15, 1458-63.

de Bloom, J., Kompler, M., Geurts, S., de Weerth, C., Taris, T. and Sonnentag, S. 2009. Do we recover from vacation? Meta-analysis of vacation effects on health and well-being. *Journal of Occupational Health*, 51, 13-25.

de Carvalho, I.A., Haour-Knipe, M. and Dehne, K.L. 2010. Migration and HIV infection: what do data from destination countries show? in *Mobility, Sexuality and AIDS*, edited by F. Thomas, M. Haour-Knipe and P. Aggleton. London: Routledge.

de Jong, K., van der Kam, S., Ford, N., Hargreaves, S., van Oosten, R. and others. 2007. The trauma of ongoing conflict and displacement in Chechnya: quantitative assessment of living conditions, and psychosocial and general health status among war displaced in Chechnya and Ingushetia. *Conflict and Health*, 1, doi: 10.1186/1752-1505-1-4.

DeHart, R.L. 2003. Health issues of air travel. *Annual Review of Public Health*, 24, 133-51.

de Wit, L., van Straten, A., Lamers, F., Cuijpers, P. and Penninx, B. 2010. Are sedentary television watching and computer use behaviours associated with anxiety and depressive disorders? *Psychiatry Research*, doi.10.1016/j. psychres.2010.07.003.

Deniz, C. and Durmusoglu, Y. 2008. Estimating shipping emissions in the region of the Sea of Marmara, Turkey. *Science of the Total Environment*, 390, 255-61.

Derudder, B. and Witlox, F. 2005. An appraisal of the use of airline data in assessing the world city network: a research note on data. *Urban Studies*, 42, 2371-88.

Derudder, B., Witlox, F., Faulconbridge, J. and Beaverstock, J. 2008. Airline data for global city network research: reviewing and refining existing approaches. *GeoJournal*, 71, 5-18.

Deshpande, A., Khoja, S., Lorca, J., McKibbon, A. and others. 2009. Asynchronous telehealth: a scoping review of analytic studies. *Open Medicine*, 3, 69-91.

Digrande, L., Neria, Y., Brackbill, R.M., Pulliam, P. and Galea, S. 2010. Long-term posttraumatic stress symptoms among 3,271 civilian survivors of the September 11, 2001, terrorist attacks on the World Trade Center. *American Journal of Epidemiology*, doi: 10.1093/aje/kwq372.

Donker, T., Wallinga, J. and Grundmann, H. 2010. Patient referral patterns and the spread of hospital-acquired infections through national health care networks, *PLoS Computational Biology*, 6, doi: 10.1371/journal.pcbi.1000715.

Dratva, J., Zemp, E., Dietrich, D.F. and others. 2001. Impact of road traffic noise annoyance on health-related quality of life: results from a population-based study. *Quality of Life Research*, 19, 37-46.

Dumurgier, J., Elbaz, A., Ducimetiere, P., Tavernier, B., Alperovitch, A. and Tzourio, C. 2009. Slow walking speed and cardiovascular death in well functioning older adults: prospective cohort study. *British Medical Journal*, 339, doi: 10.1136/bmj.b4460.

Dye, C., Lönnroth, K., Jaramillo, E., Williams, B.G. and Raviglione, M. 2009. Trends in tuberculosis incidence and their determinants in 134 countries. *Bulletin of the World Health Organization*, 87, 683-91.

Eastwood, J.B., Contory, R.E., Naicker, S., West, P.A. and others. 2005. Loss of health professionals from sub-Saharan Africa: the pivotal role of the UK. *Lancet*, 365, 1893-1900.

Edwards, P., Green, J., Roberts, I. and Lutchmun, S. 2006. Deaths from injury in children and employment status in family: analysis of trends in class specific death rates. *British Medical Journal*, 333, 119-21.

Ehntholt, K.A. and Yule, W. 2006. Practitioner review: assessment and treatment of refugee children and adolescents who have experienced war-related trauma. *Journal of Child Psychology and Psychiatry*, 47, 1197-1210.

Elbe, S. 2008. Our epidemiological footprint: the circulation of avian flu, SARS, and HIV/AIDS in the world economy. *Review of International Political Economy*, 15, 116-30.

Elkjaer, M., Shuhaibar, M., Burisch, J., Bailey, Y. and others. 2010. E-health empowers patients with ulcerative colitis: a randomised controlled trial of the web-guided 'Constant-care' approach. *Gut*, 59, 1652-61.

Ellaway, A., Macintyre, S., Hiscock, R., and Kearns, A. 2003. In the driving seat: psychosocial benefits from private motor vehicle transport compared to public transport. *Transportation Research Part F*, 6, 217-31.

Elliott, P., Toledano, M.B., Bennett, J., Beale, L., de Hoogh, K., Best, N. and Briggs, D.J. 2010. Mobile phone base stations and early childhood cancers: case-control study. *British Medical Journal*, 340, doi: 10.1136/bmj.c3077.

Elliott, S.J. and Gillie, J. 1998. Moving experiences: a qualitative analysis of health and migration. *Health & Place*, 4, 327-40.

Erickson, K.I., Raji, C.A., Lopez, O.L., Becker, J.T. and others 2010. Physical activity predicts gray matter volume in late adulthood. *Neurology*, 75, 1415-22.

Evans, A.W. 2007. Rail safety and rail privatisation in Britain. *Accident Analysis and Prevention*, 39, 510-23.

Evans, G.W. and Wener, R.E. 2006. Rail commuting duration and passenger stress. *Health Psychology*, 25, 408-12.

Evans, M.R., Shickle, D. and Morgan, M.Z. 2001. Travel illness in British package holiday tourists: prospective cohort study. *Journal of Infection*, 43, 140-7.

Ewert, A., Hollenhorst, S.J., McAvoy, L. and Russell, K.C. 2003. Therapeutic values of parks and protected areas, in *The Full Value of Parks: From Economics to the Intangible*, edited by D. Harmon and A.D. Putney. Lanham, MD: Rowman and Littlefield Publishers Inc.

Facey, M.E. 2003. The health effects of taxi driving: the case of visible minority drivers in Toronto. *Canadian Journal of Public Health*, 94, 254-7.

Farmer, A.D., Bruckner Holt, C.E.M., Cook, M.J. and Hearing, S.D. 2009. Social networking sites: a novel portal for communication. *Postgraduate Medical Journal*, 85, 455-9.

Farmer, P. 2005. *Pathologies of Power*. Los Angeles: UCLA Press.

Fennelly, K. 2007. Health and well-being of immigrants: the healthy migrant phenomenon, in *Immigrant Medicine*, edited by P.F. Walker and E.D. Barnett. Philadelphia: Elsevier.

Fidler, D. 2006. Biosecurity: friend or foe for public health governance? in *Medicine at the Border: Disease, Globalization and Security, 1850 to the Present*, edited by A. Bashford. Basingstoke: Palgrave Macmillan.

Freund, P. and Martin, G. 2001. Moving bodies: injury, dis-ease and the social organization of space. *Critical Public Health*, 11, 203-14.

Freund, P. and Martin, G. 2004. Walking and motoring: fitness and the social organisation of movement. *Sociology of Health & Illness*, 26, 273-86.

Fromme, H., Oddoy, A., Piloty, M., Krause, M. and Lahrz, T. 1998. Polycyclic aromatic hydrocarbons (PAH) and diesel engine emission (elemental carbon) inside a car and a subway train. *Science of the Total Environment*, 217, 165-73.

Gandy, M. 2008. Deadly alliances: death, disease, and the global politics of public health, in *Networked Disease: Emerging Infections in the Global City*, edited by S.H. Ali, and R. Keil. Chichester: Wiley-Blackwell.

Garshick, E., Laden, F., Hart, J.E., Rosner, B., Davis, M.E., Eisen, E.A. and Smith, T.J. 2008. Lung cancer and vehicle exhaust in trucking industry workers. *Environmental Health Perspectives*, 116, 1327-32.

Gatrell, A.C. and Elliott, S.J. 2009. *Geographies of Health: An Introduction*, London: Wiley-Blackwell.

Gatrell, C. 2010. Who rules the game? An investigation of sex-work, gender, agency and the body. *Gender in Management*, 25, 208-26.

Gauderman, W.J., Vora, H., McConnell, R., Berhane, K., Gilliland, F., and others 2007. Effect of exposure to traffic on lung development from 10 to 18 years of age: a cohort study. *Lancet*, 369, 571-77.

Gefeller, O., Tarantino, J., Lederer, P., Uter, W. and Pfahlberg, A.B. 2007. The relation between patterns of vacation sun exposure and the development of acquired melanocytic nevi in German children 6-7 years of age. *American Journal of Epidemiology*, 165, 1162-9.

Gensini, G.F., Yacoub, M.H. and Conti, A.A. 2004. The concept of quarantine in history: from plague to SARS. *Journal of Infection*, 49, 257-61.

Gesler, W.M. 1996. Lourdes: healing in a place of pilgrimage. *Health & Place*, 2, 95-106.

Gilbert, R.L., Antoine, D., French, C.E., Abubakar, I., Watson, J,M. and Jones, J.A. 2009. The impact of immigration on tuberculosis rates in the United Kingdom compared with other European countries. *International Journal of Tuberculosis and Lung Disease*, 13, 645-51.

Gill, M. and Goodacre, M. 2009. Seasonal variation in hospital admission for road traffic injuries in England: analysis of hospital statistics. *Injury Prevention*, 15, 374-8.

Gini, A. 2003. *The Importance of Being Lazy: In Praise of Play, Leisure, and Vacations*. London: Routledge.

Ginsberg, J., Mohebbi, M.H., Patel, R.S., Brammer, L. and others. 2009. Detecting influenza epidemics using search engine query data. *Nature*, 457, 1012-4.

Gleeson, B. 1999. *Geographies of Disability*. London: Routledge.

Goel, M.S., McCarthy, E.P., Philips, R.S. and Wee, C.C. 2004. Obesity among US immigrant subgroups by duration of residence. *Journal of the American Medical Association*, 292, 2860-7.

González, M.C., Hidalgo, C.A. and Barabási, A-L. 2008. Understanding individual human mobility patterns. *Nature*, 453, 779-82.

Gould, P. 1993. *The Slow Plague: A Geography of the AIDS Pandemic*. Oxford: Blackwell.

Goutziana, G., Mouchtouri, V.A., Karanila, M., Kavagias, A. and others. 2008. *Legionella* species colonization of water distribution systems, pools and air conditioning systems in cruise ships and ferries. *BMC Public Health*, doi: 10.1016/j.ajic.2009.04.285.

Grais, R.F., Ellis, J.H. and Glass, G.E. 2003. Assessing the impact of airline travel on the geographic spread of pandemic influenza. *European Journal of Epidemiology*, 18, 1065-72.

Greaves, S., Issarayandgyun, T. and Lui, Q. 2008. Exploring variability in pedestrian exposure to fine particulates (PM 2.5) along a busy road. *Atmospheric Environment*, 42, 1665-76.

Greif, M.J. and Dodoo, F.N. 2011. Internal migration to Nairobi's slums: linking migrant streams to sexual risk behavior. *Health & Place*, 17, 86-93.

Grieco, M. and Hine, J. 2008. Stranded mobilities, human disasters: the interaction of mobility and social exclusion in crisis circumstances, in *The Ethics of Mobilities: Rethinking Place, Exclusion, Freedom and Environment*, edited by S. Bergmann and T. Sager. Farnham: Ashgate.

Grove, N. and Zwi. A.B. 2006. Our health and theirs: forced migration, othering, and public health. *Social Science & Medicine*, 62, 1931-42.

Grundy, C., Steinbach, R., Edwards, P., Green, J. and others. 2009. Effect of 20 mph traffic speed zones on road injuries in London, 1986-2006: controlled interrupted time series analysis. *British Medical Journal*, 339, doi: 10.1136/bmj.b4469.

Guiver, J.W. 2007. Modal talk: discourse analysis of how people talk about bus and car travel. *Transportation Research Part A*, 41, 233-48.

Gump, B.B. and Matthews, K.A. 2000. Are vacations good for your health? The 9-year mortality experience after the multiple risk factor intervention trial. *Psychosomatic Medicine*, 62, 608-12.

Gushulak, B.D. and MacPherson, D.W. 2006. *Migration Medicine and Health: Principles and Practice*. Hamilton, Ontario: BC Decker Inc.

Hagar, C. 2009. Technology: the information and social needs of Cumbrian farmers during the UK 2001 FMD outbreak and the role of information and communication technologies (ICTs), in *The Social and Cultural Impact of Foot and Mouth Disease in the UK in 2001*, edited by Martin Döring and Brigitte Nerlich. Manchester: Manchester University Press.

Hagel, B., Macpherson, A., Rivara, F.P. and Pless, B. 2006. Arguments against helmet legislation are flawed. *British Medical Journal*, 332, 725-6.

Haggett, P. 2000. *The Geographical Structure of Epidemics*. Oxford: Oxford University Press.

Hamer, M. and Chida, Y. 2008. Active commuting and cardiovascular risk: a meta-analytic review. *Preventive Medicine*, 46, 9-13.

Handsley, S. 2009. Double clutchin', bucket tippin', juggernaut driving, truckin' time: a trucker's tale, in *Gendered Journeys, Mobile Emotions*, edited by G. Letherby and G. Reynolds. Farnham: Ashgate.

Harrington, D. and Elliott, S.J. 2009. Weighing the importance of neighborhood: a multilevel exploration of the determinants of overweight and obesity. *Social Science & Medicine*, 68, 593-600.

Hart, R. 2009. From embryo to dinosaur? A railwayman's journey, in *Gendered Journeys, Mobile Emotions*, edited by G. Letherby and G. Reynolds. Farnham: Ashgate.

Hasham, S., Majumder, S., Southern, S.J., and others. 2004. Hot-air ballooning injuries in the United Kingdom (January 1976-January 2004). *Burns*, 30, 856-60.

Herring, D.A. and Sattenspiel, L. 2007. Social contexts, syndemics, and infectious disease in northern aboriginal populations. *American Journal of Human Biology*, 19, 190-202.

Hesse, M., Tutenges, S., Schliewe, S. and Reinholdt, T. 2008. Party package travel: alcohol use and related problems in a holiday resort: a mixed methods study. *BMC Public Health*, 8, doi: 10.1186/1471-2458-8-35.

Hinchcliffe, S. and Bingham, N. 2008. People, animals, and biosecurity in and through cities, in *Networked Disease: Emerging Infections in the Global City*, edited by S.H. Ali and R. Keil. Chichester: Wiley-Blackwell.

Hiscock, R., Macintyre, S., Kearns, A. and Ellaway, A. 2002. Means of transport and ontological security: do cars provide psycho-social benefits to their users? *Transportation Research Part D*, 7, 119-35.

Hodge, D.R. 2008. Sexual trafficking in the United States: a domestic problem with transnational dimensions. *Social Work*, 53, 143-52.

Hogbin, V. 1985. Railways, disease and health in South Africa. *Social Science & Medicine*, 20, 933-8.

Hooker, C. 2006. Drawing the lines: danger and risk in the age of SARS, in *Medicine at the Border: Disease, Globalization and Security, 1850 to the Present*, edited by A. Bashford. Basingstoke: Palgrave Macmillan.

Hooker, C. 2008. SARS as a 'health scare', in *Networked Disease: Emerging Infections in the Global City*, edited by S.H. Ali and R. Keil. Chichester: Wiley-Blackwell.

Hooper, C.R. 2008. Adding insult to injury: the healthcare brain drain. *Journal of Medical Ethics*, 34, 684-7.

Horowitz, M.D., Rosensweig, J.A. and Jones, C.A. 2007. Medical tourism: globalization of the healthcare marketplace. *Medscape General Medicine*, 9, PMCID: PMC2234298.

Horton, D. 2007. Fear of cycling, in *Cycling and Society*, edited by D. Horton, P. Rosen and P. Cox. Farnham: Ashgate.

Horton, D., Rosen, P. and Cox, P. 2007. *Cycling and Society*. Farnham: Ashgate.

Hoyer, P.F. 2006. Commercial living non-related organ transplantation: a viewpoint from a developed country. *Paediatric Nephrology*, 21, 1364-8.

Hu, G., Tuomilehto, J., Borodulin, K., and Jousilahti, P. 2007. The joint associations of occupational, commuting, and leisure-time physical activity, and the Framingham risk score on the 10-year risk of coronary heart disease. *European Heart Journal*, 28, 492-8.

Hughes, R.J., Hopkins, R.J., Hill, S. and others. 2003. Frequency of venous thromboembolism in low to moderate risk long distance air travellers: the New Zealand Air Traveller's Thrombosis (NZATT) study. *Lancet*, 362, 2039-44.

Hunter, J.M. and Young, J.C. 1971. Diffusion of influenza in England and Wales. *Annals, Association of American Geographers*, 61, 637-53.

Hurling, R., Catt, M., de Boni, M., Fairley, B.W. and others. 2007. Using internet and mobile phone technology to deliver an automated physical activity program: randomized controlled trial. *Journal of Medical Internet Research*, 9, doi: 10.2196/jmir.9.2.e7.

Hygge, S., Evans, G.W., and Bullinger, M. 2002. A prospective study of some effects of aircraft noise on cognitive performance in schoolchildren. *Psychological Science*, 13, 469-74.

Idriss, S.Z., Kvedar, J.C. and Watson, A.J. 2009. The role of online support communities: benefits of expanded social networks to patients with psoriasis. *Archives of Dermatology*, 145, 46-51.

Ingold, T. 2007. *Lines: a Brief History*. London: Routledge.

Ingram, A. 2008. Domopolitics and disease: HIV/AIDS, immigration, and asylum in the UK. *Environment & Planning D*, 26, 875-94.

Inskip, P.D., Hover, R.N. and Devesa, S.S. 2010. Brain cancer incidence trends in relation to cellular telephone use in the United States. *Neuro-Oncology*, doi: 10.1093/neuonc/noq077.

Int Panis, L., de Geus, B, Vandenbulcke, G., Willems, H. and others. 2010. Exposure to particulate matter in traffic: a comparison of cyclists and car passengers. *Atmospheric Environment*, 44, 2263-70.

Interphone Study Group. 2010. Brain tumour risk in relation to mobile telephone use: results of the INTERPHONE international case-control study. *International Journal of Epidemiology*, 39, 675-94.

Jacobsen, P., Racioppi, F. and Rutter, H. 2009. Who owns the roads? How motorised traffic discourages walking and cycling. *Injury Prevention*, 15, 369-73.

Janelle, D. 1969. Time space convergence, *Annals of the Association of American Geographers*, 59, 348-64.

Jarup, L., Dudley, M.L., Babisch, W., Houthuijs, D. and others. 2005. Hypertension and exposure to noise near airports (HYENA): study design and noise exposure assessment. *Environmental Health Perspectives*, 113, 1473-8.

Jarup, L., Babisch, W., Houthuijs, D., Pershagen, G. and others. 2008. Hypertension and exposure to noise near airports: the HYENA study. *Environmental Health Perspectives*, 116, 329-33.

Jensen, A., Kaerlev, L., Tüchsen, F., Hannerz, H., Dahl, S., Nielsen, P.S. and Olsen, J. 2008. Locomotor diseases among male long-haul truck drivers and other professional drivers. *International Archives of Occupational and Environmental Health*, 81, 821-7.

Jensen, O. 2009. Foreword: mobilities as culture, in *The Cultures of Alternative Mobilities: Routes Less Travelled*, edited by P. Vannini. Farnham: Ashgate.

Jirón, P. 2009. Immobile mobility in daily travelling experiences in Santiago de Chile, in *The Cultures of Alternative Mobilities: Routes Less Travelled*, edited by P. Vannini. Farnham: Ashgate.

Joffres, C., Mills, E., Joffres, M., Khanna, T., Walia, H. and Grund, D. 2008. Sexual slavery without borders: trafficking for commercial sexual exploitation in India. *International Journal for Equity in Health*, 7, doi: 10.1186/1475-9276-7-22.

Johnson, S.T. 2009. Biosecurity: idyllic England in millennial Britain, in *The Social and Cultural Impact of Foot-and-Mouth Disease in the UK in 2001*, edited by M. Döring and B. Nerlich. Manchester: Manchester University Press.

Johnston, R., Crooks, V.A., Snyder, J. and Kingsbury, P. 2010. What is known about the effects of medical tourism in destination and departure countries? A scoping review. *International Journal of Equity in Health*, 9, doi: 10.1186/1475-9276-9-24.

Jones A.P., Sauerzapf, V. and Haynes, R. (2008) The effects of mobile speed camera introduction on road traffic crashes and casualties in a rural county of England, *Journal of Safety Research*, 39, 101-10.

Jones, C.A. and Keith, L.G. 2006. Medical tourism and reproductive outsourcing: the dawning of a new paradigm for healthcare. *International Journal of Fertility and Women's Medicine*, 51, 251-5.

Jonkman, S.N., Maaskant, B., Boyd, E. and Levitan, M.L. 2009. Loss of life caused by the flooding of New Orleans after Hurricane Katrina: analysis of the relationship between flood characteristics and mortality. *Risk Analysis*, 29, 676-97.

Juvonen, J. and Gross, E.F. 2008. Extending the school grounds? Bullying experiences in cyberspace. *Journal of School Health*, 78, 496-505.

Kakefuda, I., Stallones, L. and Gibbs, J. 2009. Discrepancy in bicycle helmet use among college students between two bicycle use purposes: commuting and recreation. *Accident Analysis and Prevention*, 41, 513-21.

Kalipeni, E. and Oppong, J. 1998. The refugee crisis in Africa and implications for health and disease: a political ecology approach. *Social Science & Medicine*, 46, 1637-53.

Kan, P., Simonsen, S.E., Lyon, J.L. and Kestle, J.R.W. 2008. Cellular phone use and brain tumor: a meta-analysis. *Journal of Neuro-oncology*, 86, 71-78.

Kaplan, M.S., Huguet, N., Newsom, J.T. and McFarland, B.H. 2004. The association between length of residence and obesity among Hispanic immigrants. *American Journal of Preventive Medicine*, 27, 323-6.

Karlsen, S. and Nazroo, J.Y. 2002. Relation between racial discrimination, social class, and health among ethnic minority groups. *American Journal of Public Health*, 92, 624-31.

Kaufmann, V. and Montulet, B. 2008. Between social and spatial mobilities: the issue of social fluidity, in *Tracing Mobilities: Towards a Cosmopolitan Perspective*, edited by W. Canzler, V. Kaufmann, and S. Kesselring, Farnham: Ashgate.

Kazmi, J.H. and Pandit, K. 2001. Disease and dislocation: the impact of refugee movements on the geography of malaria in NWFP, Pakistan. *Social Science & Medicine*, 52, 1043-55.

Kearns, R.A. 1993. Place and health: toward a reformed medical geography, *The Professional Geographer*, 45, 139-47.

Keil, R. and Ali, S.H. 2008a. SARS and the restructuring of health governance in Toronto, in *Networked Disease: Emerging Infections in the Global City*, edited by S.H. Ali and R. Keil. Chichester: Wiley-Blackwell.

Keil, R. and Ali, S.H. 2008b. 'Racism is a weapon of mass destruction': SARS and the social fabric of urban multiculturalism, in *Networked Disease: Emerging Infections in the Global City*, edited by S.H. Ali and R. Keil. Chichester: Wiley-Blackwell.

Kelly, B., Hattersley, L., King, L. and Flood, V. 2008. Persuasive food marketing to children: use of cartoons and competitions in Australian commercial television advertisements. *Health Promotion International*, 23, 337-44.

Kemp, C. and Rasbridge, L. 2004. *Refugee and Immigrant Health*. Cambridge: Cambridge University Press.

Kesselring, S. 2008. The mobile risk society, in *Tracing Mobilities: Towards a Cosmopolitan Perspective*, edited by W. Canzler, V. Kaufmann and S. Kesselring. Farnham: Ashgate.

Khan, K., Arino, J., Hu, W., Raposo, P. and others. 2009. Spread of a novel influenza A (H1N1) virus via global airline transportation. *New England Journal of Medicine*, 361, 212-4.

Kim, M-H., Subramanian, S.V., Kawachi, I. and Kim, C-Y. 2007. Association between childhood fatal injuries and socioeconomic position at individual and area levels: a multilevel study. *Journal of Epidemiology and Community Health*, 61, 135-40.

Kimball, A.M. 2006. *Risky Trade: Infectious Disease in the Era of Global Trade*. Farnham: Ashgate.

King, N.B. 2008. Networks, disease, and the utopian impulse, in *Networked Disease: Emerging Infections in the Global City*, edited by S.H. Ali and R. Keil, Chichester: Wiley-Blackwell.

Kingham, S. and Ussher, S. 2007. An assessment of the benefits of the walking school bus in Christchurch, New Zealand. *Transportation Research Part A*, 41, 502-10.

Kingma, M. 2007. Nurses on the move: a global overview. *Health Services Research*, 42, 1281-98.

Kinlen, L., Clarke, K. and Hudson, C. 1990. Evidence from population mixing in British New Towns 1946-85 of an infective basis for childhood leukaemia. *Lancet*, 336, 577-82.

Kitchin, R. 1998. *Cyberspace: The World in the Wires*. Chichester: John Wiley.

Klein, H. 1999. *The Atlantic Slave Trade*. Cambridge: Cambridge University Press.

Kleinert, M. 2009. Solitude at sea or social sailing? The constitution and perception of the cruising community, in *The Cultures of Alternative Mobilities: Routes Less Travelled*, edited by P. Vannini. Farnham: Ashgate.

Knowles, C. 2010. Mobile sociology, *British Journal of Sociology*, Special Issue, 63S, 373-9.

Knowles, R. 2006. Transport shaping space: differential collapse in time-space, *Journal of Transport Geography*, 14, 407-25.

Kortepeter, M.G., and Parker, G.W. 1999. Potential biological weapons threats. *Emerging Infectious Diseases*, 5, 523-7.

Kumarasamy, K.K., Toleman, M.A., Walsh, T.R., Bagaria, J. and others. 2010. emergence of a new antibiotic resistance mechanism in India, Pakistan, and the UK: a molecular, biological and epidemiological study. *Lancet Infectious Diseases*, 10, 597-602.

Kwan, M-P. 2007. Mobile communications: social networks, and urban travel: hypertext as a new metaphor for conceptualizing spatial interaction, *Professional Geographer*, 59, 434-46.

Kwan, M-P. and Lee, J. 2004. Geovisualization of human activity patterns using 3D GIS: A time-geographic approach, in *Spatially Integrated Social Science*, edited by M.F. Goodchild and D.G. Janelle. New York: Oxford University Press.

Labinjo, M., Juillard, C., Kobusingye, O.C. and Hyder, A.A. 2009. The burden of road traffic injuries in Nigeria: results of a population-based survey. *Injury Prevention*, 15, 157-62.

Laden, F., Hart, J.E., Eschenroeder, A., Smith T.J. and Garshick E. 2006. Historical estimation of diesel exhaust exposure in a cohort study of U.S. railroad workers and lung cancer. *Cancer Causes and Control*, 17, 911-9.

Lagarde, E., van der Loeff, M., Enel, C., Holmgren, B., and others. 2003. Mobility and the spread of human immunodeficiency virus into rural areas of West Africa. *International Journal of Epidemiology*, 32, 744-52.

Lahkola, A., Salminen, T., Raitanen, J., and others. 2008. Meningioma and mobile phone use – a collaborative case-control study in five North European countries. *International Journal of Epidemiology*, 37, 1304-13.

Landale, N.S., Gorman, B.K. and Oropesa, R.S. 2006. Selective migration and infant mortality among Puerto Ricans. *Maternal and Child Health Journal*, 10, 351-60.

Larsen, J.A. 2007. Embodiment of discrimination and overseas nurses' career progression. *Journal of Clinical Nursing*, 16, 2187-95.

Larson, A., Bell, M. and Young, A.F. 2004. Clarifying the relationships between health and residential mobility. *Social Science & Medicine*, 59, 2149-60.

Lau, C. 2008. Child prostitution in Thailand. *Journal of Child Health Care*, 12, 144-55.

Laurier, E. 2004. Doing office work on the motorway. *Theory, Culture & Society*, 21, 261-77.

Layard, R. 2005. *Happiness: Lessons from a New Science*. London: Penguin Books.

Learmonth, A. 1988. *Disease Ecology*. Oxford: Basil Blackwell.

Lebrun, L.A. and Dubay, L.C. 2010. Access to primary and preventive care among foreign-born adults in Canada and the United States. *Health Services Research*, 45, 1693-1719.

Lee, C.T., Williams, P. and Hadden, W.A. 1999. Parachuting for charity: is it worth the money? A 5-year audit of parachute injuries in Tayside and the cost to the NHS. *Injury*, 30, 283-7.

Lefebvre, C. 2009. Integrating cell phones and mobile technologies into public health practice: a social marketing perspective. *Health Promotion Practice*, 10, 490-4.

Lerer, L.B. and Scudder, T. 1999. Health impacts of large dams. *Environmental Impact Assessment Reviews*, 19, 113-23.

Lester, R.T., Ritvo, P., Mills, E.J., Kariri, A. and others. 2010. Effects of a mobile phone short message service on antiretroviral treatment adherence in Kenya (WelTel Kenya1): a randomised trial. *Lancet*, 376, 1838-45.

Levin, L. 2009. Mobility in later life: time, choice, and action in *The Cultures of Alternative Mobilities: Routes Less Travelled*, edited by P. Vannini. Farnham: Ashgate.

Likupe, G. 2006. Experiences of African nurses in the UK National Health Service: a literature review. *Journal of Clinical Nursing*, 15, 1213-20.

Lin, S., Munsie, J.P., Herdt-Losavio, M., Hwang, S.A., and others. 2008. Residential proximity to large airports and potential health impacts in New York State. *International Archives of Occupational and Environmental Health*, 81, 797-804.

Lindert, J., Schouler-Ocak, M., Heinz, A. and Priebe, S. 2008. Mental health, health care utilisation of migrants in Europe. *European Psychiatry*, 23, S14-S20.

Lindström, M. and Sundquist, K. 2005. The impact of country of birth and time in Sweden on overweight and obesity: a population-based study. *Scandinavian Journal of Public Health*, 33, 276-84.

Ling, R. 2008. *New Tech, New Ties: How Mobile Communication is Reshaping Social Cohesion*. Cambridge, MA: MIT Press.

Lippman, S., Pulerwitz, J., Chinaglia, M. and others. 2007. Mobility and its liminal context: exploring sexual partnering among truck drivers crossing the Southern Brazilian border. *Social Science & Medicine*, 65, 2464-73.

Liu, B.B., Ivers, R., Norton, R., Boufous, S., Blows, S. and Lo, S.K. 2008. Helmets for preventing injury in motorcycle riders. *Cochrane Database Systematic Reviews*, CD004333.

Long, C.R., Seburn, M., Averill, J.R. and More, T.A. 2003. Solitude experiences: varieties, settings, and individual differences. *Personality and Social Psychology Bulletin*, 29, 578-83.

Longhurst, R. 2001. *Bodies: Exploring Fluid Boundaries*. London: Routledge.

Lorant, V., van Oyen, H. and Thomas, I. 2008. Contextual factors and immigrants' health status: double jeopardy. *Health & Place*, 14, 678-92.

Lu, Y. 2008. Test of the 'healthy migrant hypothesis': a longitudinal analysis of health selectivity of internal migration in Indonesia. *Social Science & Medicine*, 67, 1331-9.

Lyons, G. and Urry, J. 2005. Travel time use in the information age. *Transportation Research Part A*, 39, 257-76.

McBeth, M. 2009. Long live the 'velorution'! Cycling, gender and the emotions, in *Gendered Journeys, Mobile Emotions*, edited by G. Letherby and G. Reynolds. Aldershot: Ashgate.

McCarthy, M. 1999. Transport and health, in *Social Determinants of Health*, edited by M. Marmot and R.G. Wilkinson. Oxford: Oxford University Press.

McConnell, R., Islam, T., Shankardass, K., Jerrett, M. and others. 2010. Childhood incident asthma and traffic-related air pollution at home and school. *Environmental Health Perspectives*, 118, 1021-6.

McEvoy, S.P., Stevenson, M.R., McCartt, A.T., Woodward, M. and others. 2005 Role of mobile phones in motor vehicle crashes resulting in hospital attendance: a case-crossover study. *British Medical Journal*, 331, 428-30.

McKelvey, A., David, A.L., Shenfield, F. and Jauniaux, E.R. 2009. The impact of cross-border reproductive care on 'fertility tourism' on NHS maternity services. *British Journal of Obstetrics and Gynaecology*, 116, 1520-3.

McLeman, R. and Smit, B. 2006. Migration as an adaptation to climate change. *Climatic Change*, 76, 31-53.

McLoughlin, P. and Warin, M. 2008. Corrosive places, inhuman spaces: mental health in Australian immigration detention. *Health & Place*, 14, 254-64.

McNeill, W.H. 1976. *Plagues and Peoples*. Oxford: Basil Blackwell.

Mackett, R.L., Lucas, L., Paskins, J. and Turbin, J. 2005. The therapeutic value of children's everyday travel. *Transportation Research Part A*, 39, 205-19.

Macpherson, A.K., Macarthur, C., To, T.M., Chipman, M.L. and others. 2006. Economic disparity in bicycle helmet use by children six years after the introduction of legislation. *Injury Prevention*, 12, 231-5.

Macpherson, A.K. and Spinks, A. 2008. Bicycle helmet legislation for the uptake of helmet use and prevention of head injuries. *Cochrane Database of Systematic Reviews*, Issue 3, CD005401.

MacPherson, D.W. and Gushulak, B.D. 2006. Balancing prevention and screening among international migrants with tuberculosis: population mobility as the major epidemiological influence in low-incidence nations. *Public Health*, 120, 712-23.

Mangili, A. and Gendreau, M.A. 2005. Transmission of infectious diseases during commercial air travel. *Lancet*, 365, 989-96.

Markel, H. 1995. 'Knocking out the cholera': cholera, class, and quarantines in New York City, 1892. *Bulletin of the History of Medicine*, 69, 420-57.

May, C., Finch, T., Mair, F. and Mort, M. 2005. Towards a wireless patient: chronic illness, scarce care and technological innovation in the United Kingdom. *Social Science & Medicine*, 61, 1485-94.

Meade, M.S. and Earickson, R.J. 2000. *Medical Geography*. London: Guilford Press.

Meade, M.S. and Emch, M. 2010. *Medical Geography*, London: Guilford Press.

Mehdi, M.R., Kim, S., Seong, J.C. and Arsalan, M.H. 2011. Spatio-temporal patterns of road traffic noise pollution in Karachi, Pakistan. *Environment International*, 37, 97-104.

Melin, A. 2008. Travelling as pilgrimage: ecotheological contributions to mobility ethics, in *Spaces of Mobility*, edited by S. Bergman, T. Hoff, and T. Sager. London: Equinox.

Miller, E., Decker, M.R., Silverman, J.G. and Raj, A. 2007. Migration, sexual exploitation, and women's health. *Violence Against Women*, 13, 486-97.

Miller, H.J. 2004. Tobler's first law and spatial analysis. *Annals, Association of American Geographers*, 94, 284-9.

Mitchell, H., Kearns, R.A. and Collins, D.C.A. 2007. Nuances of neighbourhood: children's perceptions of the space between home and school in Auckland, New Zealand. *Geoforum*, 38, 614-27.

MMWR. 2005. Public health consequences from hazardous substances acutely released during rail transit – South Carolina, 2005; selected States, 1999-2004, Centers for Disease Control (CDC), *Morbidity and Mortality Weekly Report*, 54 (3), 64-7.

MMWR. 2006. Assessment of health-related needs after hurricanes Katrina and Rita – Orleans and Jefferson Parishes, New Orleans Area, Louisiana, October 17-22, 2005, Centers for Disease Control (CDC), *Morbidity and Mortality Weekly Report*, 55 (2), 38-41.

Mokhtarian, P.L. 2005. Travel as a desired end, not just a means. *Transportation Research Part A*, 39, 93-6.

Moran, J. 2009. *On Roads*. London: Profile Books.

Mort, M., May, C.R. and Williams, T. 2003. Remote doctors and absent patients: acting at a distance in telemedicine? *Science, Technology & Human Values*, 28, 274-95.

Naci, H., Chisholm, D. and Baker, T.D. 2009. Distribution of road traffic deaths by road user group: a global comparison. *Injury Prevention*, 15, 55-9.

Naicker, S., Plange-Rhule, J., Tutt, R.C. and Eastwood, J.B. 2009. Shortage of healthcare workers in developing countries: Africa. *Ethnicity and Disease*, 19, S1-S4.

Neckerman, K.M., Lovasi. G.D., Davies, S., Purciel, M. and others. 2009. Disparities in neighbourhood conditions: evidence from GIS measures and field observation in New York City. *Journal of Public Health Policy*, 30, S264-S285.

Neri, A.J., Cramer, E.H., Vaughan, G.H., Vinje, J. and Mainzer, H.M. 2008. Passenger behaviors during norovirus outbreaks on cruise ships. *Journal of Travel Medicine*, 15, 172-6.

Newbold, K.B. 2005. Self-rated health within the Canadian immigrant population: risk and the healthy immigrant effect. *Social Science & Medicine*, 60, 1359-70.

Ng, M.K. 2008. Globalization of SARS and health governance in Hong Kong under 'one country, two systems', in *Networked Disease: Emerging Infections in the Global City*, edited by S.H. Ali and R. Keil. Chichester: Wiley-Blackwell.

Nguyen, L., Ropers, S., Nderilu, E. and others. 2008. Intent to migrate among nursing students in Uganda: measures of the brain drain in the next generation of health professionals. *Human Resources Health*, 12, doi: 10.1186/1478-4491-6-5.

Norman, P., Boyle, P. and Rees, P. 2005. Selective migration, health and deprivation: a longitudinal analysis. *Social Science & Medicine*, 60, 2755-71.

Nutton, V. 2008. *Pestilential Complexities: Understanding Medieval Plague, Medical History*. London: Supplement No. 27, Wellcome Trust Centre for the History of Medicine.

Nyanzi, S. and Bah, O. 2001. Rice, rams and remittances: bumsters and female tourists in the Gambia, in *Mobility, Sexuality and AIDS*, edited by F. Thomas, M. Haour-Knipe and P. Aggleton. London: Routledge.

Nynäs, P. 2008. Global vagabonds, place and the self: the existential dimension of mobility, in *Spaces of Mobility*, edited by S. Bergman, T. Hoff and T. Sager. London: Equinox.

O'Donnell, I. and Farmer, R.D.T. 1994. The epidemiology of suicide on the London underground, *Social Science & Medicine*. 38, 409-18.

Office for National Statistics. 2010. *Social Trends*, 40, London.

Ogilvie, D., Egan, M., Hamilton, V. and Petticrew, M. 2004. Promoting walking and cycling as an alternative to using cars: systematic review. *British Medical Journal*, 329, 763-6.

Ogilvie, D., Foster, C.E., Rothnie, H., Cavill, N. and others. 2007. Interventions to promote walking: systematic review. *British Medical Journal*, 334, doi: 10.1136/bmj.39198.722720.

Ohadike, D.C. 1991. Diffusion and physiological responses to the influenza pandemic of 1918-19 in Nigeria. *Social Science & Medicine*, 32, 1393-99.

Ohta, M., Mizoue, T., Mishima, N. and Ikeda, M. 2007. Effect of the physical activities in leisure time and commuting to work on mental health. *Journal of Occupational Health*, 49, 46-52.

Okie, S. 2007. Immigrants and health care – at the intersection of two broken systems. *New England Journal of Medicine*, 357, 525-9.

Oldenburg, M., Baur, X. and Schlaich, C. 2010. Occupational risks and challenges at seafaring. *Journal of Occupational Health*, 52, 249-56.

Oliver, L. and Kohen, D. 2009. Neighbourhood income gradients in hospitalisations due to motor vehicle traffic incidents among Canadian children. *Injury Prevention*, 15, 163-9.

Oliviera, S.A., Saraiya, M., Geller, A.C., Heneghan, M.K. and Jorgensen, C. 2006. Sun exposure and risk of melanoma. *Archives of Disease in Childhood*, 91, 131-8.

Olson, K. 1999. Aum Shinrikyo: One and Future Threat? *Emerging Infectious Diseases*, 5, 513-6.

Onyut, L.P., Neuner, F., Ertl, V., Schauer, E., Odenwald, M. and Elbert, T. 2009. Trauma, poverty and mental health among Somali and Rwandese refugees living in an African refugee settlement – an epidemiological study. *Conflict and Health*, 3, doi: 10.1186/1752-1505-3-6.

O'Riordan, D.L., Steffen, A.D., Lunde, K.B. and Gies, P. 2008. A day at the beach while on tropical vacation. *Archives of Dermatology*, 144, 1449-55.

Ory, D.T. and Mokhtarian, P.L. 2005. When getting there is half the fun? Modeling the liking for travel. *Transportation Research Part A*, 39, 97-123.

Osorio, L., Todd, J. and Bradley, D.J. 2004. Travel histories as risk factors in the analysis of urban malaria in Colombia. *American Journal of Tropical Medicine & Hygiene*, 71, 380-6.

Ost, S. 2010. The de-medicalisation of assisted dying: is a less medicalised model the way forward? *Medical Law Review*, 18, 497-540.

Ott, J.J., Winkler, V., Kyobutingi, C., Laki, J. and Becher, H. 2008. Effects of residential changes and time patterns on external-cause mortality in migrants: results of a German cohort study. *Scandinavian Journal of Public Health*, 36, 524-31.

Oudshoorn, N. 2008. Diagnosis at a distance: the invisible work of patients and healthcare professionals in cardiac telemonitoring technology. *Sociology of Health and Illness*, 30, 272-88.

Oudshoorn, N. 2009. Physical and digital proximity: emerging ways of health care in face-to-face and telemonitoring of heart-failure patients. *Sociology of Health and Illness*, 31, 390-405.

Oxford, J.S., Lambkin, R., Sefton, A. and others. 2005. A hypothesis: the conjunction of soldiers, gas, pigs, ducks, geese and horses in Northern France during the Great War provided the conditions for the emergence of 'Spanish' influenza pandemic of 1918-19. *Vaccine*, 23, 940-45.

Padilla, M.B. and Castellanos, H.D. 2010. Touristic borderlands: ethnographic reflections on Dominican social geographies, in *Mobility, Sexuality and AIDS*, edited by F. Thomas, M. Haour-Knipe and P. Aggleton. London: Routledge.

Padilla, M.B., Guilamo-Ramos, V., Bouris, A. and Reys, A.M. 2010. HIV/AIDS and tourism in the Caribbean: an ecological systems perspective. *American Journal of Public Health*, 100, 70-77.

Pagani, L.S., Fitzpatrick, C., Barnett, T.A. and Dubow, E. 2010. Prospective associations between early childhood television exposure and academic, psychosocial, and physical well-being by middle childhood. *Archives of Pediatric and Adolescent Medicine*, 164, 425-31.

Page, A.S., Cooper, A.R., Griew, P. and Jago, R. 2010. Children's screen viewing is related to psychological difficulties irrespective of physical activity. *Pediatrics*, 126, 1011-17.

Palinkas, L.A, Petterson, J.S., Russell, J. and Downs, M.A. 1993. Community patterns of psychiatric disorders after the Exxon Valdez oil spill. *American Journal of Psychiatry*, 150, 1517-23.

Pallasmaa, J. 2008. Existential homelessness – placelessness and nostalgia in the age of mobility, in *The Ethics of Mobilities: Rethinking Place, Exclusion, Freedom and Environment*, edited by S. Bergmann and T. Sager. Farnham: Ashgate.

Pardi L.A., King B.P., Salemi G., and Salvator A.E. 2007. The effect of bicycle helmet legislation on pediatric injury. *Journal of Trauma Nursing*, 14, 84-7.

Parkin, J., Ryley, T. and Jones, T. 2007. Barriers to cycling: an exploration of quantitative analyses, in *Cycling and Society*, edited by D. Horton, P. Rosen and P. Cox, P. Farnham: Ashgate.

Parkin, P.C., Khambalia, A., Kmet, L. and Macarthur, C. 2003. Influence of socioeconomic status on the effectiveness of bicycle helmet legislation for children: a prospective observational study. *Pediatrics*, 112, 192-6.

Parr, H. 2008. *Mental Health and Social Space: Towards Inclusionary Geographies*, Oxford: Blackwell.

Patterson, K.D. 1994. Cholera diffusion in Russia, 1823-1923. *Social Science & Medicine*, 38, 1171-91.

Perch-Nielsen, S.L., Bättig, M.B. and Imboden, D. 2008. Exploring the link between climate change and migration. *Climatic Change*, 91, 375-93.

Peters, J., Parry, G.D., van Cleemput, P., Moore, J. and others. 2009. Health and use of health services: a comparison between Gypsies and Travellers and other ethnic groups. *Ethnicity & Health*, 14, 359-77.

Peters, P.F. 2006. *Time, Innovation and Mobilities: Travel in Technological Cultures.* London: Routledge.

Pfeifer, G.D., Harrison, R.M. and Lynam, D.R. 1999. Personal exposure to airborne metals in London taxi drivers and office workers in 1995 and 1996. *Science of the Total Environment*, 235, 253-60.

Philbrick, J.T., Shumate, R., Siadaty, M.S. and Becker, D.M. 2007. Air travel and venous thromboembolism: a systematic review. *Journal of General Internal Medicine*, 22, 107-14.

Pilkington, P. and Kinra, S. 2005. Effectiveness of speed cameras in preventing road traffic collisions and related casualties: systematic review. *British Medical Journal*, 330, 331-4.

Pirie, G.H. 2009a. Virtuous mobility: moralising vs measuring geographical mobility in Africa. *Afrika Focus*, 22, 21-35.

Pirie, G.H. 2009b. Incidental tourism: British Imperial air travel in the 1930s. *Journal of Tourism History*, 1, 49-66.

Pooley, C., Turnbull, J. and Adams, M. 2005. *A Mobile Century? Changes in Everyday Mobility in Britain in the Twentieth Century.* Farnham: Ashgate.

Potter, S. and Bailey, I. 2008. Transport and the environment, in *Transport Geographies*, edited by R. Knowles, J. Shaw and I. Docherty. Oxford: Blackwell.

Pujazon-Zazik, M. and Park, M.J. 2010. To tweet, or not to tweet: gender differences and potential positive and negative health outcomes of adolescents' social internet use. *American Journal of Men's Health*, 4, 77-85.

Putcher, J. and Buehler, R. 2008. Making cycling irresistible: lessons from the Netherlands, Denmark and Germany. *Transport Reviews*, 28, 495-528.

Putnam, R. 2000. *Bowling Alone: The Collapse and Revival of American Community.* New York: Simon & Schuster.

Pyle, G. 1969. The diffusion of cholera in the United States in the nineteenth century. *Geographical Analysis*, 1, 59-75.

Queyriaux, B., Pradines, B., Hasseine, L., Coste, D. and others. 2009. Airport malaria. *Presse Médicale*, 38, 7-8.

Quinn, M.M., Sembajwe, G., Stoddard, A.M. and others. 2007. Social disparities in the burden of occupational exposures: results of a cross-sectional study. *American Journal of Industrial Medicine*, 50, 861-75.

Rabius, V., Pike, K.J., Wiatrek, D. and McAlister, A.L. 2008. Comparing internet assistance for smoking cessation: 13-month follow-up of a six-arm randomized controlled trial. *Journal of Medical Internet Research*, 10, doi: 10.2196/jmir.1008

Rainham, D., McDowell, I., Krewski, D. and Sawada, M. 2010. Conceptualizing the healthscape: contributions of time geography, location technologies and spatial ecology to place and health research. *Social Science & Medicine*, 70, 668-76.

Rajagopal, S. 2004. Suicide pacts and the internet. *British Medical Journal*, 329, 1298-9.

Ramirez de Arellano, A.B. 2007. Patients without borders: the emergence of medical tourism. *International Journal of Health Services*, 37, 193-8.

Ray, M. and Jat, K.R. 2010. Effect of electronic media on children, *Indian Pediatrics*. 47, 561-8.

Ray M.R., Roychoudhury, S., Mukherjee, S. and Lahiri T. 2007. Occupational benzene exposure from vehicular sources in India and its effect on hematology, lymphocyte subsets and platelet P-selectin expression. *Toxicology and Industrial Health*, 23, 167-75.

Ren, F. and Kwan, M-P. 2007. Geovisualization of human hybrid activity-travel patterns. *Transactions in GIS*, 11, 721-744.

Rettie, R. 2008. Mobile phones as network capital: facilitating connections. *Mobilities*, 3, 291-311.

Reulen, R.C., Kellen, E., Buntinx, F., Brinkman, M., and Zeegers, M.P. 2008. A meta-analysis on the association between bladder cancer and occupation. *Scandinavian Journal of Urology and Nephrology, Supplement*, 218, 64-78.

Roberts, B., Damundu, E.Y., Lomoro, O. and Sondorp, E. 2009. Post-conflict mental health needs: a cross-sectional survey of trauma, depression and associated factors in Juba, Southern Sudan. *BMC Psychiatry*, 9, doi: 10.1186/1471-244X-9-7.

Roberts, B. and Patel, P. 2010. Conflict, forced migration, sexual behaviour and HIV/AIDS, in *Mobility, Sexuality and AIDS*, edited by F. Thomas, M. Haour-Knipe and P. Aggleton. London: Routledge.

Roberts, S.E. 2002. Hazardous occupations in Great Britain. *The Lancet*, 360, 543-4.

Robinson, J. 2002. *Development and Displacement*, Oxford: Oxford University Press.

Robinson, D.L. 2006. No clear evidence from countries that have enforced the wearing of helmets. *British Medical Journal*, 332, 722-5.

Rogers, V.L., Griffin, M.Q., Wykle, M.L. and Fitzpatrick, J.J. 2009. Internet versus face-to-face therapy: emotional self-disclosure issues for young adults. *Issues in Mental Health Nursing*, 30, 596-602.

Rooney, R.M., Cramer, E.H., Mantha, S., Nichols, G. and others. 2004. A review of outbreaks of foodborne disease associated with passenger ships: evidence for risk management. *Public Health Reports*, 119, 427-34.

Rosa, H. 2003 Social acceleration: ethical and political consequences of a desynchronized high-speed society. *Constellations*, 10, 3-33.

Rosahnia, R., Narayan, K.M.V. and Oza-Frank, R. 2008. Age at arrival and risk of obesity among US immigrants. *Obesity*, 16, 2669-75.

Ross, S.M. 2008. Cognitive function following exposure to contaminated air on commercial aircraft: a case series of 27 pilots seen for clinical purposes. *Journal of Nutritional and Environmental Medicine*, 17, 111-26.

Rudant, J., Baccaini, B., Ripert, M. Goubin, A. and others. 2006. Population-mixing at the place of residence at the time of birth and incidence of childhood leukaemia in France. *European Journal of Cancer*, 42, 927-33.

Sampson, R. and Gifford, S.M. 2010. Place-making, settlement and well-being: the therapeutic landscapes of recently arrived youth with refugee backgrounds. *Health & Place*, 16, 116-31.

Santana, P., Santos, R. and Nogueira, H. 2009. The link between local environment and obesity: a multilevel analysis in the Lisbon metropolitan area, Portugal. *Social Science & Medicine*, 68, 601-9.

Schifter, J. and Thomas, F. 2010. Fantasies, dependency and denial: HIV and the sex industry in Costa Rica, in *Mobility, Sexuality and AIDS*, edited by F. Thomas, M. Haour-Knipe and P. Aggleton. London: Routledge.

Schillmeier, M. 2008. Globalizing risks – the cosmo-politics of SARS and its impact on globalizing sociology. *Mobilities*, 3, 179-99.

Schmidtke, A. 1994. Suicidal behaviour on railways in the FRG. *Social Science & Medicine,* 38, 419-26.

Schobersberger, W., Leichtfried, V., Mueck-Weymann, M. and Humpeler, E. 2009. Austrian Moderate Altitude Studies (AMAS): benefits of exposure to moderate altitudes (1,500-2,500m). *Sleep and Breathing*, 14, 201-7.

Schupp, T., Bolt, H.M., Jaeckh, R. and Hengstler, J.G. 2006. Benzene and its methyl-derivatives: derivation of maximum exposure levels in automobiles. *Toxicological Letters*, 160, 93-104.

Scott, S. and Duncan, C. 2004. *Return of the Black Death: The Worlds' Greatest Serial Killer*. Chichester: John Wiley.

Shariff, S. 2008. *Cyber-Bullying: Issues and Solutions for the School, the Classroom and the Home*. London: Routledge.

Sharma, S.N., Kumar, S., Das, B.P., Thomas, T.G. and others. 2005. Entomological indices of *Aedes aegypti* at some international airports and seaports of southern India – a report. *Journal of Communicable Diseases*, 37, 173-81.

Shaw, J. and Hesse, M. 2010. Transport, geography and the 'new' mobilities, *Transactions, Institute of British Geographers*, 35, 305-12.

Sheller, M. 2004. Automotive emotions: feeling the car. *Theory, Culture & Society*, 21, 221-42.

Shephard, R.J. 2008. Is active commuting the answer to population health? *Sports Medicine*, 38, 751-8.

Shimazono, Y. 2007. The state of the international organ trade: a provisional picture based on integration of available information. *Bulletin of the World Health Organization*, 85, 955-62.

Shu, P-Y., Chien, L-J., Chang, S-F, Su, C-L and others. 2005. Fever screening at airports and imported dengue. *Emerging Infectious Diseases*, 11, 460-62.

Silverman, D. and Gendreau. M. 2009. Medical issues associated with commercial flights. *Lancet*, 373, 2067-77.

Skinner, D. and Rosen, P. 2007. Hell is other cyclists: rethinking transport and identity, in *Cycling and Society*, edited by D. Horton, P. Rosen and P. Cox. Farnham: Ashgate.

Smith, A.D., Bradley, D.J., Smith, V., Blaze, M., Behrens, R.H., Chiodini, P.L and Whitty, C.J. (2008) Imported malaria and high risk groups: observational study using UK surveillance data 1987-2006, *British Medical Journal*, 337, doi: 10.1136/bmj.a120.

Smith, P.K., Mahdavi, J., Carvalho, M., Fisher, S., Russell, S. and Tippett, N. 2008. Cyberbullying: its nature and impact in secondary school pupils. *Journal of Child Psychology and Psychiatry*, 49, 376-85.

Sonkin, B., Edwards, P., Roberts, I. and Green, J. 2006. Walking, cycling and transport safety: an analysis of child road deaths. *Journal of the Royal Society of Medicine*, 99, 402-5.

Spiegel, P.B., Le, P, Ververs, M-T and Salama, P. 2007. Occurrence and overlap of natural disasters, complex emergencies and epidemics during the past decade (1995-2004). *Conflict and Health*, 1, doi: 10.1186/1752-1505-1-2.

Stansfeld, S.A., Berglund, B., Clark, C., Lopez-Barrio, I., and others. 2005. Aircraft and road traffic noise and children's cognition and health: a cross-national study. *Lancet*, 365, 1942-9.

Steffen, R., de Bernardis, C and Banos, A. 2003. Travel epidemiology – a global perspective. *International Journal of Antimicrobial Agents*, 21, 89-95.

Steinbach, R., Green, J., Edwards, P. and Grundy, C. 2010. 'Race' or place? Explaining ethnic variations in childhood pedestrian injury rates in London. *Health & Place*, 16, 34-42.

Stevenson, K. 2009. "Women and young girls dare not travel alone": the dangers of sexual encounters on Victorian railways, in *Gendered Journeys, Mobile Emotions*, edited by G. Letherby and G. Reynolds. Farnham: Ashgate.

Stiller, C.A., Kroll, M.E., Boyle, P.J. and Feng, Z. 2008. Population mixing, socioeconomic status and incidence of childhood acute lymphoblastic leukaemia in England and Wales: analysis by census ward. *British Journal of Cancer*, 98, 1006-11.

Stoddard, S.T., Morrison, A.C., Vazquez-Prokopec, G.M., Soldan, V.P., and others. 2009. The role of human movement in the transmission of vector-borne pathogens. *PLOS Neglected Tropical Diseases*, 3, doi: 10.1371/journal.pntd.0000481.

Stradling, S., Carreno, M., Rye, T. and Noble, A. 2007. Passenger perceptions and the ideal urban bus journey experience. *Transport Policy*, 14, 283-92.

Stradling, S. and Anable, J. 2008. Individual transport patterns, in *Transport Geographies*, edited by R. Knowles, J. Shaw and I. Docherty. Oxford: Blackwell.

Strange, C. 2006. Postcard from Plaguetown: SARS and the exoticization of Toronto, in *Medicine at the Border: Disease, Globalization and Security, 1850 to the Present*, edited by A. Bashford. Basingstoke: Palgrave Macmillan.

Strauss-Blasche, G., Ekmekcioglu, C. and Marktl, W. 2000. Does vacation enable recuperation? Changes in well-being associated with time away from work. *Occupational Medicine*, 50, 167-72.

Strauss-Blasche, G., Reithofer, B., Schobersberger, W., Ekmekcioglu, C. and Marktl, W. 2005. Effect of vacation on health: moderating factors of vacation outcome. *Journal of Travel Medicine*, 12, 94-101.

Strauss-Blasche, G., Riedmann, B., Schobersberger, W. and others. 2004. Vacation at moderate and low altitude improves perceived health in individuals with metabolic syndrome. *Journal of Travel Medicine*, 11, 300-4.

Sullivan, R., Edwards, P., Sloggett, A. and Marshall, C.E. 2009. Families bereaved by road traffic crashes: linkage of mortality records with 1971-2001 censuses. *Injury Prevention*, 15, 364-8.

Suwanvanichkij, V. 2008. Displacement and disease: The Shan exodus and infectious disease implications for Thailand. *Conflict and Health*, 2, doi: 10.1186/1752-1505-2-4.

Swaminathan, A., Torresi, J., Schlaenhauf, P., Thursky, K. and others. 2009. A global study of pathogens and host risk factors associated with infectious gastrointestinal disease in returned international travellers. *Journal of Infection*, 59, 19-27.

Tam, C. 2006. Migration and health: fact, fiction, art, politics. *Emerging Themes in Epidemiology*, 3, 1-5.

Tatem, A.J. 2009. The worldwide airline network and the dispersal of exotic species: 2007-2010. *Ecography*, 32, 94-102.

Tatem, A.J. and Hay, S.I. 2007. Climatic similarity and biological exchange in the worldwide airline transportation network. *Proceedings of the Royal Society B*, 274, 1489-96.

Tatem, A.J. and Smith, D.L. 2010. International population movements and regional *Plasmodium falciparum* malaria elimination strategies. PNAS, 107, 12222-7.

Tatem, A.J., Hay, S.I. and Rogers, D.J. 2006. Global traffic and disease vector dispersal. *Proceedings of the National Academy of Sciences of the USA*, 103, 6242-7.

Tatem, A.J., Qiu, Y., Smith, D.L. Sabot, O. and others (2009) The use of mobile phone data for the estimation of the travel patterns and imported *Plasmodium falciparum* rates among Zanzibar residents, *Malaria Journal*, 8, doi: 10.1186/1475-2875-8-287.

Tatem, A.J., Rogers, D.J. and Hay, S.I. 2006. Estimating the malaria risk of African mosquito movement by air travel. *Malaria Journal*, 5, doi: 10.1186/1475-2875-5-57.

Tatem, A.J., Rogers, D.J. and Hay, S.I. 2007. Global transport networks and infectious disease spread, in *Global Mapping of Infectious Diseases: Methods, Examples and Emerging Applications*, edited by S.I. Hay, A.J. Graham and D.J. Rogers. London: Academic Press.

Taylor, P. 2004. *World City Network: a Global Urban Analysis*. London: Routledge.

TenBrink, D., McMunn, R. and Panken, S. 2009. Project U-Turn: increasing active transportation in Jackson, Michigan. *American Journal of Preventive Medicine*, 37, S329-S335.

Thomas, F., Haour-Knipe, M. and Aggleton, P. 2010. *Mobility, Sexuality and AIDS*. London: Routledge.

Thomas, H. 1997. *The Slave Trade: The History of the Atlantic Slave Trade 1440-1870*. New York: Simon and Schuster Inc.

Ticktin, M. 2006. Medical humanitarianism in and beyond France: breaking down or patrolling borders? in *Medicine at the Border: Disease, Globalization and Security, 1850 to the Present*, edited by A. Bashford. Basingstoke: Palgrave Macmillan.

Timperio, A., Crawford, D., Telford, A. and Salmon, J. 2004. Perceptions about the local neighbourhood and walking and cycling among children. *Preventive Medicine*, 38, 39-47.

Timperio, A., Ball, K., Salmon, J, Roberts, R. and others. 2006. Personal, family, social, and environmental correlates of active commuting to school. *American Journal of Preventive Medicine*, 30, 45-51.

Tranter, P.J. 2010. Speed kills: the complex links between transport, lack of time and urban health. *Journal of Urban Health*, 87, 155-66.

Trilla, A., Trilla, G. and Daer, C. 2008. The 1918 'Spanish flu' in Spain. *Clinical Infectious Diseases*, 47, 668-73.

Tse, J.L.M., Flin, R. and Mearns, K. 2006. Bus driver well-being review: 50 years of research. *Transportation Research Part F*, 9, 89-114.

Tüchsen, F., Hannerz, H., Roepstorff, C. and Krause, N. 2006. Stroke among male professional drivers in Denmark, 1994-2003. *Occupational and Environmental Medicine*, 63, 456-60.

Tunstall, H., Pickett, K. and Johnsen, S. 2010. Residential mobility in the UK during pregnancy and infancy: are pregnant women, new mothers and infants 'unhealthy migrants'? *Social Science & Medicine*, 71, 786-98.

Turkle, S. 2011. *Alone Together: Why We Expect More from Technology and Less from Each Other*. New York: Basic Books.

UNHCR 2010. 2009 *Global Trends: Refugees, Asylum-Seekers, Returnees, Internally Displaced and Stateless Persons*, UNHCR, Geneva. Available at: www.unhcr.org/statistics.

Urry, J. 2002. Mobility and proximity. *Sociology*, 36, 255-74.

Urry, J. 2007. *Mobilities*. Cambridge: Polity Press.

Valentine, G. and Holloway, S.L. 2002. Cyberkids? Exploring children's identities and social networks in on-line and off-line worlds. *Annals, Association of American Geographers*, 92, 302-19.

van Bergen, D.D., Smit, J.H., van Balkom, A.J.L.M., van Ameijden, E. and Saharso, S. 2008. Suicidal ideation in ethnic minority and majority adolescents in Utrecht, the Netherlands. *Crisis*, 29, 202-8.

van Cleemput, P., Parry, G., Thomas, K., Peters, J. and Cooper, C. 2007. Health-related beliefs and experiences of Gypsies and Travellers: a qualitative study. *Journal of Epidemiology and Community Health*, 61, 205-10.

van den Scott, L-J. 2009. Cancelled, aborted, late, mechanical: the vagaries of air travel in Arviat, Nunavut, Canada, in *The Cultures of Alternative Mobilities: Routes Less Travelled*, edited by P. Vaninni. Farnham: Ashgate.

van Dyck, D., Deforche, B., Cardon, G. and de Bourdeaudhuij, I. 2009. Neighbourhood walkability and its particular importance for adults with a preference for passive transport. *Health & Place*, 15, 496-504.

van Wagner, E. 2008. Toward a dialectical understanding of networked disease in the global city: vulnerability, connectivity, topologies, in *Networked Disease: Emerging Infections in the Global City*, edited by S.H. Ali and R. Keil. Chichester: Wiley-Blackwell.

Vannini, P. 2009. *The Cultures of Alternative Mobilities: Routes Less Travelled.* Farnham: Ashgate.

Vannini, P. and Vannini, A. 2009. Mobility, ritual, and performance: an ethnography of parents', children's, and youth's ferry boat travel, in *The Cultures of Alternative Mobilities: Routes Less Travelled*, edited by P. Vannini. Farnham: Ashgate.

Vazquez-Prokopec G.M., Stoddard S.T., Paz-Soldan V., Morrison A.C. and others. 2008. Usefulness of commercially available GPS data-loggers for tracking human movement and exposure to dengue virus. *International Journal of Health Geographics*, 8, doi: 10.1186/1476-072X-8-68.

Viruell-Fuentes, E.A. 2007. Beyond acculturation: immigration, discrimination, and health research among Mexicans in the United States. *Social Science & Medicine*, 65, 1524-35.

Vital Wave Consulting. 2009. *mHealth for Development: the Opportunity of Mobile Technology for Healthcare in the Developing World.* Washington DC: UN Foundation-Vodafone Foundation Partnership.

Wallensten, A., Oliver, I., Ricketts, K., Kafatos, G., Stuart, J.M. and Joseph, C. 2010. Windscreen wiper fluid without added screenwash in motor vehicles: a newly identified risk factor for Legionnaires' disease. *European Journal of Epidemiology*, 25, 661-5.

Walter, S.D., King, W.D. and Marrett, L.D. 1999. Association of cutaneous malignant melanoma with intermittent exposure to ultraviolet radiation: results of a case-control study in Ontario, Canada. *International Journal of Epidemiology*, 28, 418-27.

Wang, S., Zhang, J., Zeng, X., Zeng, Y., Wang, S. and Chen, S. 2009. Association of traffic-related air pollution with children's neurobehavioral functions in Quanzhou, China. *Environmental Health Perspectives*, 117, 1612-8.

Wanvik, P.O. 2009. Effects of road lighting: an analysis based on Dutch accident statistics 1987-2006. *Accident Analysis and Prevention*, 41, 123-8.

Warfa, N., Bhui, K., Craig, T. Curtis, S. and others. 2006. Post-migration geographical mobility, mental health and health service utilisation among Somali refugees in the UK: a qualitative study. *Health & Place*, 12, 503-15.

Warren, A., Bell, M. and Budd, L. 2010. Airports, localities and disease: representations of global travel during the H1N1 pandemic. *Health & Place*, 16, 727-35.

Waskul, D.D. and Waskul, M.E. 2009. Paddle and portage: the travail of BWCA canoe travel, in *The Cultures of Alternative Mobilities: Routes Less Travelled*, edited by P. Vannini. Farnham: Ashgate.

Watters, C. 2007. Refugees at Europe's borders: the moral economy of care. *Transcultural Psychiatry*, 44, 394-417.

Webber, M.M. 1964. The urban place and the nonplace urban realm, in *Explorations into Urban Structure*, edited by M.M. Webber. Philadelphia: University of Pennsylvania Press, 79-153.

Weir, L. and Mykhalovskiy, E. 2006. The geopolitics of global public health surveillance in the twenty-first century, in *Medicine at the Border: Disease, Globalization and Security, 1850 to the Present*, edited by A. Bashford. Basingstoke: Palgrave Macmillan.

Wellman, B. 2001. Physical place and cyber place: the rise of networked individualism. *International Journal of Urban and Regional Research*, 25, 227-52.

Wen, M., Fan, J., Jin, L and Wang, G. 2010. Neighborhood effects on health among migrants and natives in Shanghai, China. *Health & Place*, 16, 452-60.

Westman, A. and Björnstig, U. 2005. Fatalities in Swedish skydiving. *Accident Analysis and Prevention*, 37, 1040-48.

Whitelegg, D. 2009. When being at work isn't work: airline cabin crew, emotional labour and travel, in *Gendered Journeys, Mobile Emotions*, edited by G. Letherby and G. Reynolds. Farnham: Ashgate.

Wiking, E., Johansson, S.E. and Sundquist, J. 2004. Ethnicity, acculturation, and self-reported health: a population based study among immigrants from Poland, Turkey, and Iran in Sweden. *Journal of Epidemiology & Community Health*, 58, 574-82.

Wild, S.H., Fischbacher, C., Brock, A., Griffiths, C. and Bhopal, R. 2007. Mortality from all causes and circulatory disease by country of birth in England and Wales 2001-2003. *Journal of Public Health*, 29, 191-8.

Williams, M.A., Soiza, R.L., Jenkinson, A.M. and Stewart, A. 2010. Exercising with computers in later life (EXCELL) – pilot and feasibility study of the acceptability of the Nintendo® WiiFit in community-dwelling fallers. BMC *Research Notes*, 3, doi: 10.1186/1756-0500-3-238.

Wilson C., Willis, C., Hendrikz, J.K., and Bellamy, N. 2006. Speed enforcement detection devices for preventing road traffic injuries. *Cochrane Database Systematic Reviews*, CD004607.

Winebrake, J.J., Cobett, J.J., Green, E.H., Lauer, A. and Eyring, V. 2009. Mitigating the health impacts of pollution from oceangoing shipping: an assessment of low-sulfur fuel mandates. *Environmental Science & Technology*, 43, 4776-82.

Witt, J. 2009. Addressing the migration of health professionals: the role of working conditions and educational placements. *BMC Public Health*, 9. doi: 10.1186/1471-2458-9-S1-S7.

Wonders, N.A. and Michalowski, R. 2001. Bodies, borders, and sex tourism in a globalized world: a tale of two cities – Amsterdam and Havana. *Social Problems*, 48, 545-71.

Woodcock, J. and Aldred, R. 2008. Cars, corporations, and commodities: consequences for the social determinants of health. *Emerging Themes in Epidemiology*, 5, doi: 10.1186/1742-7622-5-4.

Wright, D., Flis, N. and Gupta, M. 2008. The 'brain drain' of physicians: historical antecedents to an ethical debate, c. 1960-79. *Philosophy, Ethics, and Humanities in Medicine*, 3, doi: 10.1186/1747-5341-3-24.

Wylie, J. 2005. A single day's walking: narrating self and landscape on the South West Coast Path. *Transactions, Institute of British Geographers*, 30, 234-47.

Ybarra, M.L. and Mitchell, K.J. 2008. How risky are social networking sites? A comparison of places online where youth sexual solicitation and harassment occurs. *Pediatrics*, 121, 350-7.

York, D. 2008. Medical tourism: the trend towards outsourcing medical procedures to foreign countries. *Journal of Continuing Education in the Health Professions*, 28, 99-102.

Zagury, E., le Moullec, Y. and Momas, I. 2000. Exposure of Paris taxi drivers to automobile air pollutants within their vehicles. *Occupational and Environmental Medicine*, 57, 406-10.

Zook, M.A. and Brunn, S.D. 2006. From podes to antipodes: positionalities and global airline geographies, *Annals, Association of American Geographers*, 96, 471-90.

Zylberman, P. 2006. Civilizing the state: borders, weak states and international health in modern Europe, in *Medicine at the Border: Disease, Globalization and Security, 1850 to the Present*, edited by A. Bashford. Basingstoke: Palgrave Macmillan.

Index